YOUR BODY DOESN'T FEEL RIGHT
BUT YOU DON'T KNOW WHY

IT'S NOT IN YOUR HEAD

By Dr. Efrat LaMandre, PhD, FNP-C

DEDICATION

To GG

Who saw it in me years before I ever did

To My 3 Monkeys

For making it so easy to be a mom

Edited by Lil Barcaski and Linda Hinkle

Published by: GWN Publishing

www.GWNPublishing.com

Cover Design: Kristina Conatser, Cayla Raymundo and Kehrt Monroe Etherton

Print ISBN: 979-8-9859746-5-2
Kindle ISBN: 979-8-9859746-4-5

CONTENTS

IT'S NOT IN YOUR HEAD

WHAT MADE YOU PICK UP THIS BOOK?

If you're one of the lucky people who wakes up feeling phenomenal every day of your life, this book is not for you.

If you spring out of bed every morning, feeling great after a solid night of sleep, ready to tackle the day, this book is not for you.

If you are pain free, clear-minded, have no belly issues, and are rarely sick or anxious, I am so very happy for you but please, do us both a favor

PUT THIS BOOK DOWN.

(or, give it to someone who isn't as lucky as you)

Now, if you're still here, rest assured, you are in the right place, and you have the right book.

I'm going to assume that you are not feeling so great all the time. That's okay. You are not alone and more importantly as you will see, what you are feeling **IS NOT IN YOUR HEAD**.

I wrote this book because, after years of practice, I realized that there are just too many patients who are not being heard. Too many patients who are either told in one way or another that its "in their head" or not given options of how to treat their issues.

In fact, the patients I have worked with over the years tend to fall into one of these categories. Which one are you? (P.S. you can be in more than one.)

1. You're maybe 40 to 60ish in age and have been healthy most of your life. You take pretty good care of yourself, keep up with some of your annual physicals and screenings. You exercise some and eat a mostly healthy diet.

   But now, it feels like the wheels are starting to fall off the bus. There are days you're unexpectedly dragging along, your energy is low, you're not sleeping well. You'd just like to feel like your "old self."

   You're feeling a little more than just dragging. You have these weird symptoms—maybe your belly is off, or you have frequent headaches, heart palpitations—you've been to a whole bunch of specialists, and they say, "it's your hormones" or "it's your age" or some variations of "it's in your head." But you know there must be a better way.

2. You've seen your primary care provider and got a diagnosis. Now you're on a recommended medication that you may need to stay on for the rest of your life. Maybe you have diabetes, high blood pressure, cholesterol or maybe you've been given medications for depression and anxiety. You're not happy about taking meds, and you're wondering if there is any other way to manage all this.

3. You've been given a more complicated diagnosis, have seen multiple specialists, each one to manage your various issues, but no one is connecting the dots or talking about the root cause of all these ailments. You want answers to questions, but you're not even sure what questions to ask.

4. None of the aforementioned applies to you. In your case, you feel like you are doing the right things, but you know the future

is coming for you. You want to find the best ways to optimize your healthcare and prevent illness for as long as possible.

Like I said, if you are in one of these categories—this book is for you. I wrote this book to give you a different approach to these issues. I want to equip you with the right questions to ask so that you can get the answers you are looking for. Of course, you can always work with me and my team at The Knew Method (at the end of the book, we will tell you more about that) but this book is about give you what you need to figure it out **ON YOUR OWN**.

Fair warning though, **PROCEED WITH CAUTION**.

WHAT I'M GOING TO TEACH YOU WILL REQUIRE CHANGE. IN FACT, WE CALL OUR PATIENTS—"GAME CHANGERS."

So, once again, I implore you—if you are not ready to make change and be the **GAME CHANGER** in your own life—**PUT THIS BOOK DOWN**!

If you are still here let's get started. See you in Chapter 1.

CHAPTER 1:

MY "WHY"

THIS IS A GOOD CHAPTER, BUT IT WON'T AFFECT YOUR HEALTH IF YOU SKIP IT

WHY DID I WRITE THIS BOOK?

Let's be honest, nothing motivates us more than when things become personal. Everything changes when a problem hits home. When you or someone you love is in jeopardy, you will move heaven and earth to find a solution. I learned this lesson firsthand when my wife was suffering, and we couldn't find an answer.

What I learned on that journey with my wife profoundly changed my thinking about medical care. It changed my life and my career, and now I want to change the lives of people like you who need some actual answers to why you're feeling like you do.

MY PERSONAL BACKGROUND (IN CASE YOU WANT TO KNOW WHO I AM AND WHY YOU SHOULD LISTEN TO ME):

This may surprise you. My first degree was in English literature. Life takes you on some twists and turns, doesn't it? Despite my love for books and words, I found my healthcare calling was much stronger, so many years later, I found myself in the medical field. I got my nursing degree and started working on a medical/surgical floor (that's what we call a typical hospital floor). Before long, I shifted to the high drama of the ER and then moved on to a trauma ER. Yes, it's a lot like the TV shows you've seen and, yes, I saw it all. Gunshot victims, lost limbs, heart attacks—things stuck in places they shouldn't be—you name it—these eyes have seen it, in fact, I had a front row seat.

The ER is about stabilizing patients and then either discharging them or moving them to the next level of care. Over time, I realized I wanted to do more than patch someone up and send them onward. I found that I had a desire to be more involved in the process of getting people back to their optimal health and make the calls when it came to the patient's path to getting better. So, I went back to school to become a Family Nurse Practitioner.

I chose family medicine because it allowed me to work with all ages, and it also meant that I could be the medical provider for entire families. It is wonderful to take care of so many varied patients, and there is also something magical about taking care of several generations of the same family.

My first job out of school was in Orthopedic Pain Management; that was a great learning experience about peoples' aches and pains. Then, I got the opportunity to work in a family practice in a lower income area, and I jumped at the chance. The patients I met there were dealing with a lot more than their health issues. They faced tough financial and socioeconomic challenges. A lot of times, they were uninsured. This meant our patients didn't have access to many tests or treatment options. This made all the clinicians in that practice so much better because we had to rely on our clinical skills to diagnose and treat. I'm grateful for the time I spent there and that experience.

I realized within a year that I wanted to do this on my own and use what I had learned to provide medical care in my own community, so I opened EG Healthcare (I'm E, and my wife is G). I bought my own building, hired a great staff, and quickly began to see success as a primary care provider. The practice is growing, the reviews are amazing, and we consistently exceed industry standards. I am very active in the community through my involvement in local events and fundraisers. Now we serve over 20,000 patients, I sit on the Hospital Board of Trustees, and I'm the President of the York Nurse Practitioner Association. (So basically, I'm fancy now.)

But ...here's the clincher. In my first few years, I had a few patients that I just couldn't figure out how to help. The patients who came in and just felt "off." The tests I ran indicated that they were "fine." I sent them to various specialists who also said they were "fine." Everyone (including me) kept telling them they were "fine," but they weren't fine. So, I admit it, I was like many of the medical providers you met in your life—I blamed it on their age, their hormones, sometimes, I even said it was "in their head." (I'm sorry). This was not out of malice—it's just what we learned in school—find the disease and treat it. If there is no sign of disease, the patient is "fine." I had no idea that there might be more.

Until it hit home. At this time, my wife was experiencing some health issues and what I learned next changed my thinking.

THE STORY OF E AND G(INA) AND HOW IT BECAME PERSONAL

So, I told you I was working in the ER earlier in my career. That's where I met Gina. We were working in the trenches in that same ER. (Sort of like the plot of a cheesy Lifetime movie, right?). At that time, I was a nurse, she was a P.A., and I didn't listen to any of the orders she gave me in the ER. (Not much has changed—just kidding, honey.)

When I met Gina, I found out that she was a vampire. She wasn't the cool kind of vampire that is immortal and moves fast but she was a vampire in that she could not go out in the sun.

Before joining the medical profession, Gina was a Division One softball coach and a nationally rising star. Her job was to travel around the country, especially during the spring and summer months, to recruit and coach athletes. Obviously, this required her to be outside—a lot. She began to get mysterious and very painful rashes on her face and be out of commission for days. It took her years to get properly diagnosed because the reaction would happen days after exposure, so it made it difficult to connect the dots.

It turned out that she had something called polymorphous light eruption (PMLE). That's a fancy way of saying she was allergic to the sun, (and yes, that's a real thing). So, I like to tell people I was married to a vampire, which may be an exaggeration but it's still a fun thing to say.

Since her entire job depended on her working outdoors, her career became impossible. She decided to go to school to become a P.A. and stay out of the daylight. *Cue E and G meet at the ER*. I always say that if she hadn't had this disease, we might never have met, so I thank the universe and its mysterious ways.

By the time I met her, she had been dealing with this for a few years and was adjusted to the lifestyle it created. I had to adjust too. We only ventured out late afternoons and evenings, and I got used to living on the non-sunny side of the street.

Maybe you can relate to this. Most people, and the people who love them, are resilient. When they don't feel well or get diagnosed with something, they learn to accommodate. The people with the achy knees stop running, the people with the stomach issues take some Tums, and the people who are allergic to the sun, just don't go out. You figure it out, you make do. You accept your fate. Right? Sound familiar?

It usually takes something else, a second diagnosis, the next medication, or feeling worse before you start looking for answers.

That's exactly how it was for us. We learned to adjust our lifestyle to Gina's first disease, but then something changed. Suddenly, we found ourselves searching for a new set of answers when it became clear that she was dealing with something new.

Gina developed a second autoimmune disease. It's very common that if you have one autoimmune issue, you will likely develop another. (You will find out why in Chapter 3, so feel free to skip over there). That's because the root of the problem was never addressed. In Gina's case, she developed severe psoriasis located on her limbs but also on her hands and bottoms of her feet. It was awful. Her feet would bleed, her skin would crack, and she couldn't button her shirts or open a jar without debilitating pain.

That's when we started looking for answers. We went to several skin specialists who advised us that she would need medication. We tried some of those medications, and they would work ... temporarily, but the issues would always come back. Clearly, this wasn't a path we wanted to stay on long-term. What we wanted were real answers as to why this was happening. Remember, at this point, we are both in the medical field, many of our friends were in the medical field, so we had access to everything but still couldn't get the answers we needed.

One of our friends suggested a doctor who practiced functional medicine. Truthfully, we had never even heard of functional medicine, but we thought, why not give it a try but we also totally rolled our eyes at the same time because we figured that this probably wouldn't work. We met the doctor, and he did these weird labs that we had never learned about in our schooling. He concluded that the answer was to radically change her diet. In fact, he insisted that what Gina was eating was causing her skin issues. This was insanity. Nothing we ever learned in school connected food to psoriasis, let alone to PMLE. This guy was clearly off his rocker.

His suggestion was ridiculous; my wife was already a healthy eater. She was athletic, never ate junk food, in fact, she was a vegetarian! How can this guy suggest that her diet was off? Well, it turned out that Gina's "healthy" diet *was* causing her skin issues. As a vegetarian, many of her food choices were corn and soy heavy. The testing that we did showed that she was sensitive to corn and soy!

SIDE NOTE: I am not against a vegetarian diet at all, I'm also not saying corn and soy is bad for everyone—I'm just sharing Gina's results here.)

After changing her diet and beginning to use the supplements he recommended, the results were amazing and fast. Within weeks, her psoriasis cleared up, the pain was gone, and we began to realize that she was also no longer as sensitive to the sun. Soon enough, we found that we could go out any time of the day. That's not to say that Gina could spend a lazy day on the beach in mid-summer, but she could go out and participate in normal daytime activities. *Vampires no more!*

Watching this medical provider work, seeing the tests he used, and learning about his methods, I felt as if I was seeing a whole new way of thinking about medicine. I knew that I had to explore this and bring this to my practice. I thought, *why don't I try some of this with my own patients?*

Of course, this led me back to school. I began my education at The Institute of Functional Medicine and then I decided to go all in and pursue my Ph.D. in Integrative Medicine. What I found interesting is that the people I studied with were all medical professionals, each of whom had come to functional medicine in a similar way as I had. Like me, they had a strong connection to someone who was suffering from something that could not be treated by conventional medicine. It was personal for them the way it was for me. When you or someone you love is suffering, your wife, parent, a child, you desperately want them to get better. You want the answers. These other medical providers had come to the same realization that I had—that there was a better way, and they wanted to learn everything they could for their patients and their loved ones.

As I continued to learn more about functional medicine, I realized that this was not only for people who already had a diagnosis like my wife. I realized that all those people who came in telling me that they "weren't feeling well" were, in fact, **NOT WELL**. The reasons that the test(s) kept telling me they were "fine" is because they were the **WRONG TESTS**.

Let me explain, in conventional medicine, we run tests that help us find diseases. If there is no disease, you are fine. End of story. See you next year. Conventional medicine is not set up to find things that are "cooking." It turns out that there are tests we can run to let us know that something is "up" and can help validate the patients who know something is off. It also turns out that if we intervene and start making some lifestyle changes, we can stop the disease from happening, and if we already have the diagnosis, we can improve the outcome!

I got fired up by this realization and that's why and how I created *The Knew Method*, which is my signature process to empower my patients to finally realize that their symptoms are not in their head and help them get better and feel great again. I will get into all of that soon.

CHAPTER 2:

YOU'RE NOT ALONE

WHAT YOU AND MANY OTHERS ARE FEELING

So, let's talk about what you may have experienced so far. If you're like some of my patients, maybe you've picked up this book because you are feeling off, not optimal. Perhaps you have seen medical providers of several different disciplines and have been told things like, "you're just stressed," or "you're just getting older," or "if you lose weight, you'll feel better," or "you're just experiencing the usual symptoms of menopause, hormones," or ... maybe ... "it's all in your head!"

Or maybe you're already on two or three medications, and you're not crazy about taking them. You're wondering if there's a better solution for you.

Or maybe you're "fine" now but want to know how to optimize things.

If you picked up this book, it's likely that you haven't gotten the answers that you are looking for or at least not the ones that have helped you feel any better. There are real reasons for the way you are feeling, and there are ways to feel better! We're going to talk about those reasons in depth.

THE "I-DON'T-FEEL-GOOD" SPECTRUM

Let's start to figure out where you are in your health journey. If you're like the range of patients that come to me, you've likely experienced one of these scenarios. If you read the introduction, I said there were four kinds of people who would benefit from reading this book. Now, I want to talk about what each of those four groups of people have likely experienced when they sought answers from their medical provider. Does any of this sound familiar?

Medical Experience #1: "I don't feel good-itis."

You're not feeling in tip-top shape like you used to. Maybe you're tired more than usual or worse, you find yourself dragging through the day trying to keep up with kids, parents, work, life. Your energy is low. Perhaps you're not sleeping as well. Maybe you're having mild anxiety or feeling depressed. You go to your medical provider and when you say, "I don't feel good. I don't feel like myself," the typical response might be something like, "Your labs are fine, you're fine. You're just looking at middle-age, you're not going to feel the way you did in your twenties and thirties. It's par for the course."

You leave with your questions unanswered. Basically just ... "deal with it." So, now not only do you feel like something is wrong and don't know what, but you feel unheard or under the suspicion that you're making it all up (#crazy).

You have what I refer to as "I don't feel good-itis."

Medical Experience #2: Take the meds, and we will see you in a few months.

You're told you have something treatable, like diabetes, high-blood pressure, cholesterol, and you are given a prescription. Or maybe you've been given medication for depression and anxiety.

With this diagnosis, your primary care provider is doing the right thing by giving you medication for the health problem you've been diagnosed as having. But no one has had a conversation with you to discuss can we do this alternatively? No one has spoken to you about other options.

Again, just take the meds, and we will see you in a few months

Medical Experience #3: Nothing is connected to anything.

You've been given a more complicated diagnosis. You might have an autoimmune issue, thyroid, Crohn's, or something that was harder to diagnose and is harder to treat. You may have flareups. You've seen multiple specialists, each one to manage a different body part. The rheumatologist is managing your autoimmune disease. The GI specialist is managing your belly, the dermatologist is managing your skin and so on.

No one is offering you a conversation about the root cause of all these ailments. And no one is connecting any of these conditions to each other.

Medical Experience #4: If it ain't broke, don't fix it.

Maybe you don't fall into any of the first three experiences. You are seeking to find a way to optimize your healthcare and prevent illness. But when you have an experience in the medical world, there is no conversation about optimization, and there are minimal conversations about prevention other than watch your weight and keep exercising.

What these four patient experiences have in common is that—from people who are seeking to optimize their health to those who have a difficult diagnosis—everyone is in the same boat. No one is being offered solutions to get healthy or feel better.

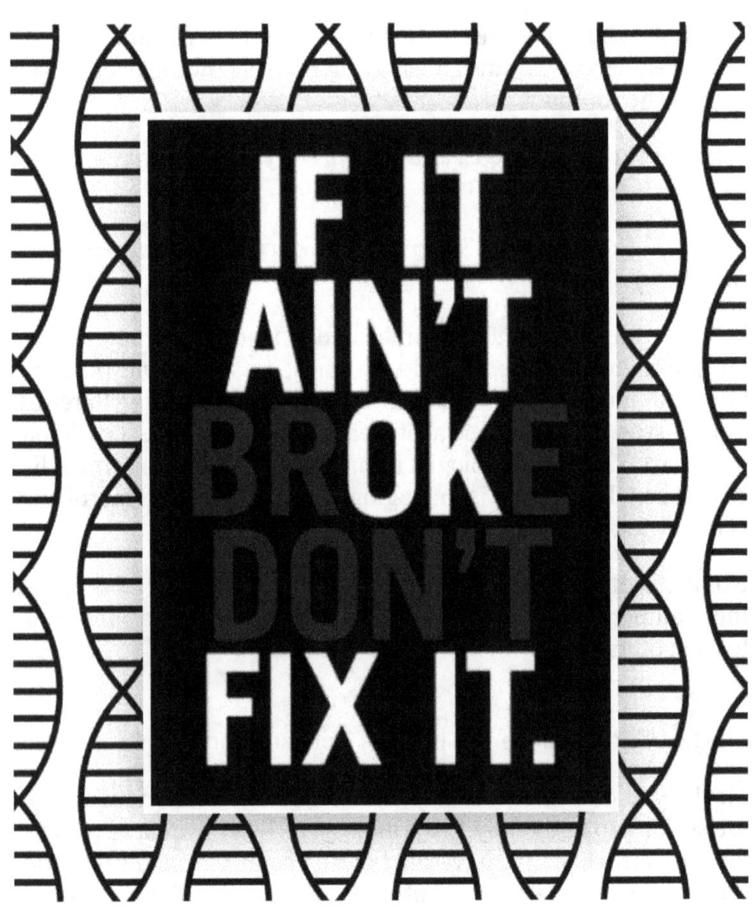

YES, YES, THAT'S ME! SO, WHAT DO I DO?

Well, at this point, if you're like most people, you start grabbing at straws. You begin Google searches to find what your symptoms might be telling you. You ask well-meaning people in your life, who say they have solutions, to share their experiences and "knowledge." But let's face it, once you start down the rabbit hole that is Google, it just becomes more confusing and overwhelming. If you Google your symptoms, you can find answers on a slippery slope ranging from "it's nothing" to "you're dying." No matter what the diagnosis is they also tell you "be sure to talk to your medical provider"—thanks Google, I already tried that!

You all know what I'm talking about. If you keep going down that road, you will spiral into the abyss of possibilities. But I get it. We all want answers when we don't feel well, and you haven't gotten them.

STOP GOOGLING FOR ANSWERS AND KEEP READING

Look, it's fair to say that the wellness world is jam packed with information and misinformation. So many people are suffering and don't know the root cause of their pain. Everywhere you turn, you hear about a quick fix, a new diet, or a miracle powder that's going to make it all go away. Let me make it clear right now, that's not what we're going to talk about in this book. I have no miracles to offer, just common-sense protocols to follow. Nothing that I suggest is a "quick fix." Once again, let me tell you—if you are looking for a quick fix—its time to give this book to someone else.

My goal in writing this book is to empower you to become the game changer in your own life and find your own actual path to good health. As I mentioned before, we call the patients we work with our game changers. Whether you work with us or someone else, we want you to become that game changer for YOUR life.

SO, HOW DOES IT WORK?

I've learned a lot on my journey, and I created a method. I'm going to share that method with you. I'm going to share a lot of the information I learned. Once you've read this book, you're going to be able to see some ways to improve your own health. But, even if you can't or don't want to go it on your own, you'll be better equipped to ask the right questions and work with a provider who can help you.

If, after you read the book, you want to work with me, great. Reach out to my office, and we can tell you how. Or, if there's a functional medicine provider in your area that you want to work with, once you're done reading this, you'll have a lot more insight on where to start, what to ask for, and what labs and tests you may need. I just want you to know how to get the answers you are looking for and start making the changes that will make you feel better.

A WORD ABOUT PRIMARY CARE AND YOUR HEALTH

I mentioned a few times above that your primary care providers may not be giving you the answers you want but I want to say for the record that I still love primary care and primary care providers. My first practice, EG Healthcare is and will always be, primary care, because is a critical part of our health. We need more PCPs in this country. Their role is critical for every patient. A good primary care physician will serve as your hub in the healthcare maze. A good PCP will help you with prevention, screening and know when it's time to escalate care. **DON'T LEAVE YOUR PRIMARY CARE PROVIDERS**!

At EG Healthcare, we continue to offer annual visits and screenings as well as diagnose and treat as necessary. Primary care, like most of conventional medicine, is about just that—searching for a diagnosis and treating it. You test, find the diagnosis, and treat. If it's too complicated, you send the patient to a specialist, and they will test, diagnose, and treat. THIS IS NOT WRONG! You better believe that I will use conventional medicine if I need to, and so should you!

The problem is that the system is not designed to help people who don't have a diagnosis but just don't feel well. It is also not designed for people who want a different way of treating their current diagnosis. For that, you need a functional medicine provider. You should use both approaches in tandem. Ideally, your functional medicine provider and your PCP should communicate if necessary and come up with a combined approach. It is usually the patient that is the go-between between the two providers—and that's okay too. Just be sure that you are utilizing both types of approaches as necessary. It is NOT an either/or choice that you need to make; it should be both.

Chapter 3 through 6 get a little technical. They explain the reasons why you don't feel good and the reason behind how to fix it. If you want to skip all this and go right to the protocol, go to Chapter 7. Then, give the book to the next person who needs it.

CHAPTER 3:

OKAY, YOU PROMISED TO TELL ME WHY I DON'T FEEL GOOD

SO, WHAT IS IT?

HERE IS THE NUMBER ONE COMMON DENOMINATOR

No, it's not a deep dark secret that I am about to reveal, but it may be something that has never been explained to you. I am willing to bet that no one has suggested this as the root cause of your health issues. Nearly all the symptoms that the people who come to me have in common, what puts them in the state of "I don't feel good-itis" comes down to one main factor—***inflammation***.

The truth is, whatever it is that you're feeling—your achy joints, your belly discomfort, your allergies, your food sensitivities, it all starts with inflammation. And it's not the same for everyone because not everyone experiences the same symptoms or level of pain and discomfort. Inflammation is a spectrum that ranges from the state of "I don't feel good-itis" without any diagnosis all the way to diseases and chronic illness.

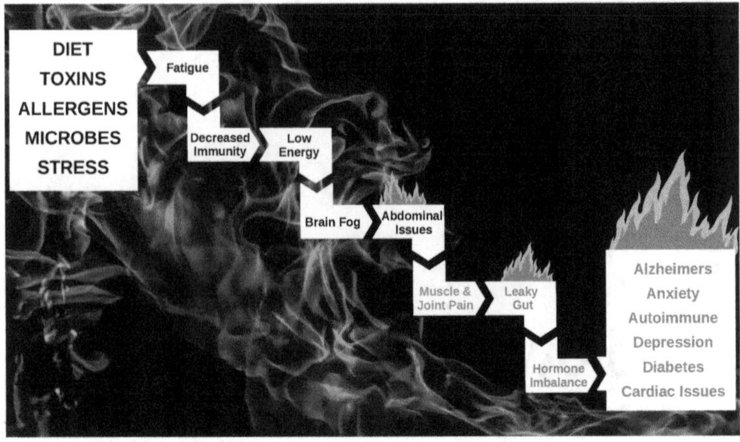

Look at this chart. On the top left, you will see that there are certain factors in our lives—what we eat, how we sleep, our stress, things we are exposed to—trauma, medications, infections—that can cause inflammation in our bodies. That inflammation affects each person differently. For some, it will create a feeling of unwell and for others, it will cause disease. You can be anywhere on this spectrum, and all of it is caused by inflammation.

What you can see from this chart is that, given enough time and enough inflammation, all the symptoms that you have will lead to disease.

Let's be clear, not all inflammation is bad!

Inflammation is important, and we need it to survive because inflammation is a vital part of the immune system's response to injury and infection. It is the body's way of signaling the immune system to heal and repair damaged tissue as well as defend itself against foreign invaders such as viruses and bacteria.

But *chronic* inflammation is not good. It's a problem, and when that exists, it leads to much bigger problems.

Good inflammation

Let's say we fall and hurt ourselves; when that happens, the body recognizes that we have had an injury and inflammation helps get blood to the damaged area. The area swells (becomes inflamed), it does this because it is bringing white blood cells and other types of cells to repair the area. The swelling is part of the healing process. In a few days, the swelling goes down, and the area heals. This type of temporary inflammation happens every time you injure or strain yourself; it gets worse for a few days, and then it improves. We call this acute inflammation or short-term inflammation.

Inflammation is the body's response to microbial, metabolic, or physical injury. It is a necessary part of healing.

Chronic Inflammation

The problem starts when inflammation in the body is prolonged, then it is called chronic inflammation, which wreaks havoc on the body. It can find harbor in different parts of the body—the belly, the joints, the brain, and it creates the state of "I don't feel good-itis." This kind of inflammation stays with you all the time and, unless the inflammation is controlled or reversed, it will get worse.

Over time, chronic inflammation will lead to disease. Depending on where the inflammation is, it will affect that specific organ. Inflammation in the brain causes Alzheimer's. Inflammation in the skin causes rashes; in the lungs, it can cause respiratory issues, and it can cause nearly anything from general joint pain to creating a cascade effect that leads to more serious inflammation and diseases like coronary heart disease and cancer.

If you don't believe that inflammation is a big issue, consider how many anti-inflammatories are sold in this country. Aspirin, ibuprofen, naproxen, more than 30 billion tablets are sold per year over the counter, and even more are written at prescription strength. None of these drugs treat the underlying cause, but they sure do point to the fact that we are inflamed.

Inflammation is a symptom of almost every disease, and it often makes matters worse for the person suffering that disease. Any disorder that ends with an "itis" is inflammatory. That is why I call it "I don't feel good-itis." Arthritis, rheumatoid arthritis, and dermatitis for example, are all inflammatory diseases.

So, you should now have an understanding that inflammation is the underlying cause of most diseases, and it's the core message of this book. If you can start to see how much this affects your health, you can start to work toward "feeling better." Conventional medicine already recognizes some disease as an inflammatory disease. Allergies, asthma, cardiovascular disease, and arthritis for example are considered inflammatory diseases, but the truth is, the list doesn't end there.

Almost every disease starts with inflammation. It is insidious, and it brews in the body way before disease becomes noticeable. By the time you have an official diagnosis, inflammation has already done some serious damage. You might start out with a little indigestion after you eat something spicy. That progresses into more difficulty digesting a wider variety of foods. This can escalate into stomach pains, diarrhea, or constipation. The inflammation will begin to cause other issues in the body such as joint pains or skin irritations.

We have met patients who are on different places along the inflammation spectrum ranging from people having low energy and some indigestion, or those can't perform at the gym like they used to, along with those who struggling with fatigue and brain fog. Others are in so much pain they can't get out of bed or can't walk to the mailbox to get their mail without debilitating pain. Some can't sleep, and when sleep doesn't come, they become depressed and exhausted, causing additional health issues that tend to spiral downwards.

When we don't feel good, we are inflamed. We don't have to wait for this inflammation to become a disease. We must recognize that inflammation is happening and stop it before it becomes a disease or worsens the disease we already have. There are things that tell us there is inflammation in our bodies, we refer to them as markers, and they let us know something is wrong.

WHAT CAUSES INFLAMMATION IN OUR BODIES?

What causes inflammation is different for each person. Let's go over some of the ways that inflammation can get into our body:

1. Physical injury

Getting injured is impossible to avoid. All throughout our lives, we're subject to falling, bruising, and getting cuts and scrapes that cause temporary inflammation. Multiple injuries, however, can create chronic inflammation.

Avoiding over straining is important. The weekend warrior who works out intensely or engages in a lot of strenuous activities on days off puts strain and stress on their body. They might sustain injuries repeatedly, which then creates inflammation.

Being mindful and avoiding injuries is important. Look at what happens to football players and boxers after multiple injuries. Their bodies never get the chance to recover before the next injury and the next. The injuries are cumulative, and with most contact sports, even when wearing helmets or head gear, the head is in danger of being struck over and over. Head injuries can cause brain inflammation in much the same way any overuse activities can cause inflammation in the system. Once the system is dealing with chronic inflammation, we can see symptoms in other areas of the body.

2. Psycho-emotional

Mental and emotional stress promotes inflammation and reduces immunity. It also often leads to sleep issues which exacerbates inflammation. So, this creates a loop—inflammation messes with our sleep, then being sleep-deprived, it gives us more inflammation. This is a hard loop to break out of. Much like repeated injuries, stress adds up like building blocks, creating more and more inflammation.

Again, that inflammation that started off from emotional stress can now affect our physical bodies and create physical symptoms and diseases.

When our bodies are burdened by life events, our environment, and the chronic stress that can build in our systems, this is referred to as our "Allostatic load." When our life challenges create a stress level that is more than we can cope with, we wind up with *allostatic overload*. We see studies all the time suggesting that stress is the cause of several of our health problems and diseases. In fact, stress plays a part in 50 to 70 percent of all physical illnesses, and in extreme cases, it can lead to death. That's why stress reduction is so important when we are trying to reduce inflammation and illness.

3. Infections

Infections cause our body to have reactions to fight them off. Those reactions are how we stay alive every time we get sick. Remember to fight an infection, we need inflammation, and we need that when we get the occasional flu or cold. The problem starts when the inflammation doesn't go away.

For some people, it means repeated infections. These are the people who get colds frequently. They are constantly battling an illness, which means they are constantly in inflammation. This is a cycle; people with weak immune systems will get frequent colds but these frequent illnesses are in turn weakening their system because of the inflammation.

Then, there are people who have a chronic illness and may not even be aware of it. A classic example are people who have Lyme for years and may not even know it. Your body is actively fighting a pathogen in the background, which is creating this constant continuous stream of inflammation. As I said, this can go on for years and patients may have various symptoms in their joints, their skin, and/or the brain and not know that the source is the inflammation caused by the pathogen.

Other chronic infections that can follow this pattern are the Epstein-Barr Virus (EBV) and h pylori. These pathogens create constant inflammation in the body and can create a constellation of symptoms for years before the actual issue is found and treated.

4. Environmental Toxins

Our bodies are affected by our environment. We may be exposed to environmental issues such a smoke, mold, chemicals, and heavy metals. There are toxins in the air, and even in the water in many communities. Workplaces are often filled with toxic chemicals, and there is no way to avoid them for people who need to work in those environments.

Surprisingly, some people can clear these chemicals more effectively than others. Partly, this is genetics and partly it is about overload and how much our system can clear. We're all built differently. So, for some people, environmental toxins can lead to severe illnesses, while for others, there may be mild or even no symptoms at all. This might make it harder for doctors to see the fact that environmental toxins are part of the problem when the results can be different in different people. For those people who cannot clear the toxins, the buildup creates inflammation in the system, which in turn causes symptoms and disease.

5. Diet

The Standard American Diet (SAD diet) is pro-inflammatory. The SAD diet (and the acronym *really* fits) generally has servings that are too large, with plenty of high-fat foods, high-sugar desserts and drinks, red meat, refined grains, and high-fat dairy products. It generally lacks fruit, vegetables, whole grains, fish, nuts, and seeds. It has been linked to obesity, heart disease, cancer and a host of other diseases.

> **NERD ALERT:** A high intake of sugar and refined grains increases blood sugar and insulin levels which increases inflammation which, in turn, increases something called free radicals, which are molecules in our body that contain oxygen with an uneven number of electrons. The uneven number allows them to react easily with other molecules, meaning they can cause large chain chemical reactions in the body. That's

called oxidation. Oxidative stress happens when there is an imbalance between free radicals and antioxidants in your body.

When functioning properly, free radicals can help fight off pathogens, which lead to infections. This is why it is important to keep the proper balance of free radicals and antioxidants in the body. Excess free radicals can begin damaging fatty tissue and proteins in the body, which can lead to many types of diseases.

TRANSLATION: *We all know by now that all these carbs and sugars can lead to diabetes. But on the way to diabetes is years of insulin resistance. This is what people call "Pre-diabetes." This state causes so much inflammation in the body that basically this means that your high-carb diet could be causing your knee pain.*

The SAD diet is also high in something called Omega 6. We will go into Omega 6 and Omega 3 later in this book, but for now you need to know that Omega 3 is great, and Omega 6 isn't that great. We need both, but we need to have a ratio that is high in Omega 3 and low in Omega 6. I'm sure you guess by now that Omega 6 causes inflammation. So, those French fries and chicken nuggets could be causing your aches, pains, and skin issues.

YOU CANNOT REMOVE INFLAMMATION FROM YOUR BODY IF YOU ARE EATING INFLAMMATORY FOODS ALL DAY. This is why you will see in Chapter 4 that we always start with diet when we try to remove inflammation.

6. Allergies and food sensitivities

People are suffering with allergies more now than ever, and allergy symptoms have become more severe. While no one has been able to prove exactly why this is happening, it seems likely that the answer lies in the fact that we are exposed to more chemicals in our diet, in our water, and in our air than ever before. This creates an endless loop of being inflamed. An inflamed system is more likely to be triggered by an allergen and more likely to have a severe reaction.

It's not natural for us to be allergic to nature itself. Why are we allergic to pollen, ragweed, flowers, even bees, cats, or dogs? This was not always the case in the history of humanity. It's becoming more and more common, so we need to look at what's changed over the centuries, and food and environmental toxins seem to be at the core.

More people are living in cities today in crowded conditions, and there is more industry, more vehicles on the road and all of this leads to more toxicity in our air quality. There are more chemicals, and even plastic found in our food than ever in history. No matter what the causes are, it is undeniable that we are seeing more people who are suffering from allergies than ever before. When you see allergies, you are seeing inflammation, so the bottom line is, there are more people who are experiencing inflammation than ever before. And, like all the other loops we described, it goes like this—inflammation makes us more likely to be allergic, and the allergic reaction causes more inflammation and around it goes.

Food sensitivities have also been on the rise. Food sensitives are different than food allergies Most of us are familiar with food allergies. We think of examples like, I eat a banana, I get a rash. That is a histamine reaction, which is why we take antihistamines when we realize we are allergic to something. Food sensitivities are harder to pinpoint and harder to test.

Food sensitivity creates a situation where you are unable to break down certain foods, thereby affecting your digestive system and you may experience gas pains, diarrhea, or other stomach discomfort. The reaction to food sensitivity may be more delayed, and it may take more than one exposure to realize that you are sensitive to a certain food or food group. More people than ever are sensitive to things like gluten and dairy. We've become used to feeling bad after we eat; we think that there may be something wrong with our belly when in fact it's your body telling you that it's not happy with the food it's getting.

7. GI Permeability - Leaky Gut

In a normal healthy GI, there is a barrier of tight junctions that has an important job. It allows the good stuff—nutrients and water—in and blocks access to certain substances from going into the blood stream that should not be able to get in. But for some people, that barrier is loose, and certain protein or amino acids get through. When those substances get through, the body reacts to it as it would to a foreign invader, and this process causes inflammation. We are going to talk at length about leaky gut later in the book. It's a very important subject and affects many people, but for now you just need to know that it is another source of inflammation in the body.

8. Being Overweight

Fat cells secrete their own inflammation, which creates a cascade of more inflammation. This is part of the reason why being overweight can lead to health problems. Being overweight leads to higher risk of being diabetic, which is an inflammatory disease. You find yourself in a never-ending cycle, excess weight causing inflammation, inflammation causing diseases, including diabetes, which causes more inflammation. There is no way to get off the merry-go-round. This simmers over the years, leaving you just one big ball of inflammation.

Inflammatory disorders start out mild and eventually become more serious and difficult to treat. For example, over time, mild gastritis can lead to ulcers, esophagitis, and cancer. Athletic injuries sustained over time can lead to arthritis. It is easier to reverse and treat the inflammation than the disease.

In addition, diseases come in groups. If you don't treat the inflammation, it will keep attacking different body parts. That is why my wife started out with PMLE and then got psoriasis. This explains why someone will have thyroid issues and diabetes, etc. It's because each time, we are treating the disease (medication for thyroid, medication for diabetes) but we are not treating the cause, which is inflammation. Treat the root cause, and you treat all the diseases at once.

Which disease you will have depends largely on your genetics. If you have a family history of thyroid issues and you lead a proinflammatory lifestyle, the inflammation will result in thyroid disease whereas your neighbor with the same diet may end up with heart disease or diabetes.

But you don't have to wind up with the same health issues and diseases as your family history might dictate. You are not destined to be sick just because of your genetics. Become a gamechanger and change your health destiny!

INFLAMMATION AFFECTS EVERYTHING.

› **THE BRAIN AND NERVOUS SYSTEM**—brain fog, depression, anxiety, issues with concentration, and ultimately, Alzheimer's
› **DIGESTIVE TRACT**—stomach issues, constipation, diarrhea, heartburn
› **LIVER AND KIDNEYS**—lymphatic (detox) swelling, rashes overall discomfort
› **PANCREAS**—sugar regulation, prediabetes, diabetes, weight gain
› **ENDOCRINE SYSTEM**—hormones, thyroid adrenal, thinning hair, dry skin and weak nails, menstruation, low sex drive
› **MUSCLE, JOINTS, AND CONNECTIVE TISSUE**—muscle pain, joint stiffness, fibromyalgia, achiness
› **IMMUNE SYSTEM**—when overactivity becomes autoimmunity, it can impact every system, causing Hashimoto's, multiple sclerosis, rheumatoid arthritis, and skin conditions

And, yes, you can have inflammation in more than one area at a time. Your leaky gut might be causing the pain in your knees, and, at the same time, you may be experiencing skin conditions, even psoriasis.

TESTING FOR INFLAMMATION

If you do get tested for inflammation, you will want to understand what the labs are telling you.

CRP Testing:

Testing for the protein made by your liver will let us know if your CRP level is high and the protein is being sent into your bloodstream in response to inflammation.

The CRP test measures how much CRP is in your blood allowing the detection of inflammation. The test is a general marker for inflammation and lets your healthcare provider determine if your symptoms are related to an inflammatory or a non-inflammatory condition and helps narrow down the possible causes of the inflammation. This test gives us what is called a non-specific marker. It won't tell us exactly where the inflammation is coming from in the body. Is it your belly or your joints? This test can't pinpoint that. It just lets us know that you're in a state of inflammation.

ESR Testing:

ESR is an acronym for Erythrocyte Sedimentation Rate. The test will tell us how quickly red blood cells settle in the bottom of a test tube over a period of one hour. It is a test to measure inflammation. If the red blood cells settle faster, it means that your ESR is higher, and there is inflammation or infection.

Be aware that even if you have these lab tests done and the results are negative, it doesn't mean you don't have inflammation; it just means that this test did not capture it. Having a positive result confirms inflammation, but having a negative result doesn't mean you are not inflamed.

You might not "feel good" for a long time before any markers show up. Markers help us, but the markers will only start after you've been inflamed for a long time. This is why we tend to find these autoimmune issues later on in life. It takes a while for them to show up.

BOTTOM LINE: Don't assume you are off the hook if your labs don't determine anything negative.

CHAPTER 4:

HOW DO I GET RID OF THE INFLAMMATION?

WE START WITH THE GUT

"OKAY, SO I GET IT! I'M INFLAMED, BUT HOW DO I KNOW WHERE TO START?"

It's a little confusing. I just told you that there are all different things that can cause inflammation. So, how do you know if you have an infection? Or maybe it's an environmental toxin like mold? Or maybe it's a food sensitivity? I didn't even mention the possibility that it might be your hormones! And ... we all know that if you Google any of these, you probably have at least half of the symptoms associated with any of these issues. So, where should you start?

The answer is easy—always start with the **GUT**. At The Knew Method, we have a phrase we use, "First, we clear the weeds, then we plant the trees." Before we even start considering any testing for mold, hormones, or food sensitivities, we always fix the gut first. You will see me say this several times in the book. We do this for two reasons. 1) It keeps things simple. For most of our patients, cleaning up the diet solves most of the symptoms without any additional testing or cost. Super simple. Fix the gut, fix the issue. 2) For those patients who are a little more complex, we STILL fix the gut first because any treatment we may need for infection, mold or other toxin will require a strengthened immune system, which means a healthy gut. I won't even consider treating for toxins unless my patient has already changed their diet and healed their gut.

Treating a patient for mold or Lyme is very taxing on the liver, and no provider in their right mind would start treating you for those things if your gut isn't healed. Mold detox, for example, uses binders which really taxes your liver. Imagine starting that kind of protocol on someone whose liver is still working hard processing a bad diet. It will be too much. Even hormones shouldn't be started on someone whose diet isn't on point because many times the diet itself can fix the hormones without any additional help.

Trust me, doing it in this order will save you time and money and will get you feeling better faster.

So, for all of you reading this book, try this part first before you do any fancy tests that you may not need; it's free and simple. (I didn't say it was easy ☺.) If, after you have implemented the changes, you are STILL not feeling well, that's when we dive into the vortex of other possible causes and we will get into that in Chapter 7.

Okay, I think you've got it now; no matter what, start at the gut!

Before I start explaining how to repair the gut, there is an important topic we need to discuss and that is Leaky Gut and to do that, we need to understand a little bit about something called "Gut Barriers."

GUT BARRIERS

When we eat a plate of food, whether it comes from a restaurant, a food truck, or even if we cook it ourselves, it all goes to the same place, the gut. By "gut," which is not really a medical term, we mean the entire GI system from your mouth to your anus. This entire system is lined with barriers, and this barrier system plays an extremely important job in keeping you safe.

This barrier is working all the time, even when you're asleep. It has two big jobs: 1) it gets all the nutrients out of our food and into our system 2) it blocks toxins from getting into the system. It's basically like a selective bouncer at a nightclub.

Only the VIP nutrients get in, and anyone who isn't invited to the event can't get in. This system is constantly working; in fact, it takes 40% of our energy at any given time to do that. It's amazing how our system works all the time to get the job done. Give that bouncer a raise!

WHAT IS LEAKY GUT?

Leaky gut occurs when something is wrong with that barrier. The bouncer is getting a little less selective and starts letting some undesirables in. Understand that this happens on a molecular level. There are no actual leaks or holes you can see, not even in a colonoscopy or endoscopy.

TIGHT JUNCTIONS

On the molecular level, these barriers have what we refer to as "tight junctions," which are like gates. The job of these "gates" are to allow nutrients in and allow toxins out, so they can be expelled from the body.

If our tight junctions become too loose or begin to stay open for too long, we have "intestinal permeability," which is the fancy way of saying leaky gut. When we have intestinal permeability, it means that harmful things that are not supposed to be in our system can escape into our bloodstream.

So, these harmful things can get into our body. Why is that important?

Well, when our body sees something foreign, it responds. That's how our immune system works. That's how we manage a cold or a virus. The body sees something it does not recognize as safe. And it attacks it. It does this by creating an inflammatory response to rid the body of this foreign invader. If all goes well, the body wins, and the patient feels better, and everything goes back to baseline.

When we have leaky gut, certain food proteins get in the system, and the body starts to treat it like a foreign object and starts to create an inflammatory response. This seems appropriate until you realize that this will now happen at every single meal. Now, you have created chronic inflammation.

If you are having GI (gastrointestinal) symptoms like belly pain, bloating, or discomfort after you eat, that's a big neon sign telling you that you may have leaky gut. However, by understanding this inflammatory cascade, you can recognize that even if you don't have GI symptoms, it doesn't mean you can eliminate the possibility of a leaky gut. The inflammation isn't just in your belly. You can have inflammation in other areas of your body. So, for example a person with leaky gut may end up with skin issues even if their belly feels fine. Remember, inflammation affects every system in your body. Here are some examples of what leaky gut can do to your system.

Okay, so maybe I have leaky gut but why do you care so much? Because leaky gut can affect just about every system in your body. Here are some examples of what leaky gut can do to your system.

AUTOIMMUNE DISEASE: There are many studies now that link leaky gut to autoimmune disease. So, if you have an autoimmune disease, or if it's in your family history, it is critical that you fix your leaky gut.

Let's dig a little deeper here. "Auto" means self, so an autoimmune disease equates to your body's immune system is attacking itself.

As we said, people with a leaky gut have an immune system that is reacting to food proteins, and from there, it's just a hop, skip, and a jump before the body starts attacking its own proteins. This is called molecular mimicry.

That's when your body reacts to a protein because A) it is very similar to protein and B) the most classic example of this is with gluten and thyroid. If the body is reactive to the gluten protein, it will often be reactive to the thyroid protein. This means that the same process the body uses to attack the gluten is now going to attack the thyroid. So, every time we eat gluten, the body thinks we are asking it to attack both the gluten and the thyroid. One of the first things we recommend to people who have thyroid issues is to cut the gluten out of their diets for this very reason.

Another way that leaky gut can affect autoimmune disease is through inflammation. The inflammation created during this food reaction process is now chronic inflammation. If we are eating the foods that cause inflammation every meal, we have constant, chronic inflammation. This inflammation now starts to activate your entire system, it doesn't just stay in the belly. If you have an autoimmune issue in your genes, this inflammation will now turn itself on. If your family history includes diabetes, which is an autoimmune issue, your inflammatory response will likely turn on your genetic predisposition to diabetes.

If your genetic predisposition is to Alzheimer's, your inflammatory process is going to turn on the Alzheimer's gene.

The good news is that **IF YOU CONTROL THE INFLAMMATION, YOU MAY BE ABLE TO PREVENT ALL OF THIS.**

Using diabetes as an example, even if your grandfather had diabetes, it doesn't mean you are going to automatically become diabetic. You still must **EAT** your way to diabetes. Even if diabetes is in your genetics; if you don't eat the carbs, you won't have diabetes. But, if you do have a genetic predisposition to diabetes, an inflammatory diet full of carbs and sugars will turn that gene on real quick.

This is true for many of the genes you carry. Of course, there are certain genes (like eye color) that we have no way to change. But, other genes, such as autoimmune genes don't have to be turned on (or expressed). Inflammation plays a role in the expression of these genes. So bottom line, **KEEP YOUR INFLAMMATION LOW**!

HORMONES: Leaky Gut can affect your hormones in so many ways.

One classic example is polycystic ovary syndrome (PCOS). With a leaky gut, you may see an increase in insulin resistance, and you will then see a rise in your testosterone level. Most women, throughout their lives, will have a testosterone level anywhere from 0-40 ng/dl, with 40 being the highest testosterone level a healthy female should have. Women with PCOS will have levels from about 60 to 100. The point of this example is just to show you that how you eat can affect your hormones. While we are on the topic of testosterone, do you know that a high-carb diet for men can increase their estrogen and lower their testosterone? These are just two examples. So, here's the bottom line, how you eat will affect your hormones. This explains why I don't recommend starting any hormone replacement therapy until you first fix your diet.

STOMACH: A leaky gut, of course, can affect the gut. It's kind of obvious—it's in the name—but we still need to take a moment to look at what it does. Inflammation in the belly can cause a whole host of issues that range in severity.

A leaky gut and its associated inflammatory response can start by causing mild discomfort, bloating, and gas, but over time, that inflammation can cause more serious diseases. A lot of people are familiar with gastroesophageal reflux disease, better known as GERD, which is fancy speak for acid reflux. Initially, you may just take a few TUMS to help with the reflux or try not to overdo the red sauce. But did you know that over time, if GERD is allowed to continue, it will eventually wear out your esophagus and can cause esophageal cancer? So, something as simple as GERD or acid reflux, if left unchecked, can lead to esophageal cancer. This is a classic example of the Inflammation spectrum; it can cause anything from mild discomfort to cancer depending on how long and how severe the inflammation is.

There are so many examples like that in the GI system. Minor inflammation can cause something called IBS (inflammatory Bowel Syndrome) and intense inflammation over time can cause a very serious condition called (IBD), also known as either Crohn's or ulcerative colitis, which is a very serious and a debilitating GI disease of chronic inflammation in your digestive tract.

SKIN: You might be surprised to know that the skin and the belly are connected. If you have something going on with your skin, you probably have something going on with your belly. Eczema, acne, psoriasis, rosacea, are often related to problems in your belly. Prescription creams might help flareups, but it is not likely they can truly resolve your skin issues. Many times, this has something to do with the microbiome, which I will explain later in this chapter. For now, what you need to know is that until you fix your belly, your skin issues won't be resolved either.

MENTAL HEALTH: Here is another surprise. Your stomach issues can affect your mental health! Anxiety and depression can be traced to gut health, and something called the gut-brain axis. You know that feeling you get in your belly when you're nervous or stressed? That's the brain talking to the belly. Well, guess what? It talks back. There is a two-way communication between your brain and your gut (the axis). While medications are certainly needed and can help quell symptoms of depression and anxiety, it would behoove anyone suffering with mental health issues to consider healing their gut issues to maximize this gut-brain axis communication and maybe, over time, reduce their medication.

MUSCLE AND JOINT PAIN: It's clear that some muscle and joint pains may be secondary to an injury, a trauma, or over exercising—we know this. But what is amazing is that many of the aches and pains we've grown accustomed to or blamed on things like old age, or our weight, are a result of inflammation, which as you can see by now, often starts in the belly. Fix the belly, fix the joint pain.

THYROID: As I mentioned earlier. A leaky gut and thyroid conditions go hand in hand. If your gut is a mess, it can affect your thyroid because of the inflammatory response I discussed earlier. What's even more maddening is that when your thyroid is not functioning at full capacity, it can lead to inflammation, which can cause a leaky gut. It's a crazy inflammation-thyroid loop.

It should be very clear by now that leaky gut and inflammation affects everything and that no matter what is going on with you—you should start with fixing your diet and healing your belly.

HOW AND WHEN DID THIS HAPPEN TO ME? AKA, HOW DID I GET A LEAKY GUT?

To get the answer to that, we need to talk about the microbiome and dysbiosis.

Microbiome

The microbiome consists of trillions of living microbes in your gut. Inside the world that lives in your belly is a delicate balance of good and bad bacteria. The good and bad must be equally balanced. Obviously, you shouldn't have too much bad bacteria, but you shouldn't have too much good either. A diverse amount of good and bad bacteria creates a thriving microbiome, which helps regulate your digestive system.

When this is messed with, we have a fancy word for it—dysbiosis.

What causes dysbiosis?

A) ***One big cause is the use of antibiotics.*** You already know that I am not against antibiotics; I will prescribe antibiotics to a patient when needed, but I do everything I can to avoid prescribing them if possible. (P.S. You don't need antibiotics for a little cold or sniffles; it does more harm than good.)

B) ***Non-steroidal anti-inflammatory drugs*** (NSAIDs) like Advil, Motrin, and aspirin, taken over time, will mess with your gut. We take these a lot in America. You know the drill. You're having joint and muscle pain, so you pop a few of these at least once or twice a day. They help relieve the pain, so they must be okay, right? Wrong. These NSAIDS start messing with the microbiome, which causes leaky gut, which is causing your joint pain and around and around we go.

C) ***Stomach bugs and viruses are a factor.*** You may have experienced something like, "Ever since I had (fill- in-the-blank bug or flu) I haven't been the same." That's because those bugs mess with your microbiome and have started a leaky gut issue. It's not in your head; it's in your gut.

D) ***Stress messes with your microbiome.*** Physical and mental stress become chronic stress and create an imbalance. Toxins, like mold, can also be a stress on the delicate balance of the microbiome.

However, the number one thing that messes with your microbiome is ...

E) ***Your diet.*** Sugar, alcohol, artificial sweeteners, dairy, and gluten are all contributors to dysbiosis. This is just the short list of foods that can mess with your belly. Some people have issues with legumes, grains, and nightshades as well.

Sorry, there is no way of escaping it. You must change your diet to feel better.

OKAY, BUT ARE THERE ANY TESTS FOR LEAKY GUT?

Yes. I want to take just a moment to talk about a test that was popular about a decade ago. It's called the Lactulose Mannitol Ratio. In this test, the patient would drink lactulose and mannitol, which are types of sugar. If the sugars were found in the urine samples, the conclusion was that the patient had leaky gut. This is an old-school test that is not considered accurate anymore. I only mention it because you might see it on Google, and I wanted to let you know **NOT** to get this one.

Currently, we do antibody testing. You've no doubt heard the term antibody at this point, but let's take a moment to define the word again. When our body sees something as a foreign object, it fights it off. Once it's done fighting, it creates a memory of it so that it knows how to fight it again next time. This memory cell is the antibody. So, when we have an antibody to something, we have been exposed to that thing. We have now discovered that there are certain antibodies that are specific to leaky gut. If we see them in our blood, we know they shouldn't be there, and its presence indicates a leaky gut.

TESTING FOR LEAKY GUT

So, we learned that when the barriers in our stomach lining are weak and our tight junctions become loose, we will experience a leaky gut. Like I said, it will affect everything.

But how do we know if we have a leaky gut? How do we test for it?

START BY NOT TESTING.

What?

Yes, there are tests for leaky gut, and I'm going to explain that in a bit, but I told you, I'm trying to save you time and money. You don't need fancy tests. The simplest way to test for leaky gut is to clean up your diet and see if it helps. Use the 4R protocol that I will describe in the next section. Just do it and if it helps, you're done! No need to test. **THERE IS NO DOWNSIDE TO THIS.** There are no negative side effects to eating better. You have no risk of hurting yourself by choosing broccoli or a baked sweet potato over greasy French fries and pizza.

Start the protocol and see if you start to feel better. If you do, guess what?

Yup, you got leaky gut!

This is a similar concept that I use for my patients who come to me and want to figure out if they are lactose intolerant. I suggest that, instead of going through a series of tests, they try taking dairy out of their diet and see if they feel better. If they remove milk, cheese, and other dairy products from the equation and stop having the symptoms they've been experiencing, they are very likely lactose intolerant.

Done and done.

The following is a list of indicators for leaky gut:

NERD ALERT (feel free to skip this section):

LPS Lipopolysaccharides:

Lipopolysaccharides (LPS) are large molecules found in bacteria. They are endotoxins, which means they can produce a strong immune response and inflammation. If the body was exposed to LPS, it will make an antibody to it. So, when we do a blood test, and we see antibodies to LPS, we know the body was exposed. The way these LPS molecules get into the bloodstream is through a leaky gut

Occludin and Zonulin:

Occludin and Zonulin are proteins of the tight junctions found between epithelial cells of the intestinal barrier. These proteins are gatekeepers of the body, allowing only small amino acid nutrients to pass into the bloodstream. When tight junction proteins are functioning properly, they prevent large molecules from crossing the intestinal barrier into the bloodstream, where they can elicit an immune response.

As the gut becomes inflamed and breaks down during leaky gut, these proteins enter the bloodstream. Once they enter the system, the body will make antibodies to it. Like with LPS, if we see antibodies to occludin or zonulin, it means they have entered the blood stream, and the only way they could do that is if there is a leaky gut. So, one way to evaluate leaky gut is to test for elevated zonulin-occludin antibodies.

Actomyosin:

Actomyosin is a smooth muscle protein found throughout the body. It lines the gut, and all the proteins together form cables called the "Actin Network." This cable network crosses the inside of the gut and connects the tight junctions. They help the tight junctions open and close to allow small amino acid nutrients to get into the bloodstream as needed.

Just like the other tests above, we shouldn't see antibodies to Actomyosin. If we see antibodies to the Actin Network in the blood, it's another indication of intestinal destruction. Actomyosin antibodies indicate gut damage is severe enough to break through the cells, not just open the spaces between cells. This type of damage takes longer to repair.

THE 4R PROTOCOL

SO, HOW DO WE FIX LEAKY GUT? THE 4R PROTOCOL

Let me make this clear. I did not invent this protocol. This is a very well-known protocol in Functional Medicine. It's been around for years and IT WORKS.

It's a four-step process.

The 4Rs stand for **REMOVE, REPLACE, REINOCULATE,** and **REPAIR**

Try it out. If you feel better, stop reading and give the book to the next person who is suffering.

Remove:

Remove anything that is injuring that barrier in your gut. That includes certain foods but also certain pathogens.

Let's start with foods. There are certain foods that simply must go for everyone. Broadly speaking, that means junk food. We've discussed at length, that inflammatory foods are going to cause leaky gut, which will allow more proteins into circulation.

For a person without leaky gut, 98% of ingested food antigens are blocked from entering circulation. But for people with leaky gut, the more antigens that get in, the more inflammation is created.

So, this may mean removing not only the high-fructose corn sugar and the refined sugars, but also gluten, dairy, corn, and soy. This is not a one-size-fits-all for every patient. There are also some people who will have to eliminate grains, legumes, and eggs. Some of these things will be eliminated forever, and some will only have to be eliminated for a few weeks and may be able to be reintroduced later.

For those of you who work with us or another provider, you will be able to create a customized plan but for those of you who just want to try it, I will give you a basic guide in Appendix 1. I also recommend Intermittent Fasting to my patients and for more details on that, see Appendix 2 as well.

SIDE NOTE: Removal also means removing pathogens. If you have H pylori or any other type of bacteria, that will need to be addressed and removed. Again, we don't have to go down that road at this time because I want you to be able to jump in and try the protocol, but just know that "removal" may also mean removing pathogens if needed.

Replace:

Just as important as it is to take troublesome foods OUT of your diet is ensuring that you have good foods IN your diet. It's not enough to just eliminate food; you also must put the good stuff in to help heal your belly and your entire system. A common mistake that people make when they try to repair their gut is that they find one or two things they like, and they eat those every day. They think that since these things are on the "good" list—eating them every day should work. The patients sometimes feel great at first because they eliminated so many of the foods that were bothering their system but over time, this type of diet can create more problems in your microbiome. The microbiome needs diversity. Venture out and try new vegetables and fruits that you haven't tried before. Eat different colors. Fruits and veggies have different colors because of something called phytonutrients, which are chemicals produced by plants that give them their color. Foods with phytonutrients have antioxidant and anti-inflammatory benefits. So, make sure you "eat the rainbow."

SIDE NOTE: Removing the offending agents and adding good quality food should be enough, but some of you may also need to replace essential ingredients needed for digestion and absorption. These are digestive enzymes and stomach acid (hydrochloric acid) for proper digestion and are vital to help us get the nutrients we need out of food. Enzymes and acid break food down so that we can get the nutrients out of the food we eat. If digestive enzymes are depleted, the whole process is off. Digestion become slow, and the protein sits in the stomach instead of getting digested. Many of us do not have enough enzymes because of years of poor diet, medication, disease, and aging. As a result, some of my patients will need supplements of digestive enzymes as part of the "Replace" phase of the protocol. This part of "Replace" may require working with a functional medicine provider.

To conclude, when we are talking about the second **"R" REPLACE**, first and foremost, we mean replacing with good quality food of many colors and nutrients. At times, we may also need to replace some digestive enzymes, but this is not always necessary.

Reinoculation:

Earlier in the book, we expressed the need for a balance of good and bad bacteria in the body. To inoculate, in microbiology, means to put an organism into something. In this case, we want to put good bacteria into the gut.

Another word for good bacteria is "probiotics." Remember, we need to have a balance of good and bad bacteria. We've already discussed that when this balance is off, it is called dysbiosis. Dysbiosis happens for many reasons, however, one common reason is antibiotic use. Antibiotics kill the bad bacteria causing an infection, but at the same time, they also kill the good bacteria. This creates an imbalance that we have also discussed called dysbiosis.

Another cause of dysbiosis is the Standard American Diet, which doesn't promote good bacteria growth. So, if you eat a typical western diet, and have taken antibiotics in your life, you likely need to fix your dysbiosis with some type of probiotics.

One way to do this is to take a supplement. Supplements are full of these bacteria are called probiotics.

There are also foods that have good bacteria in them. Anything that is fermented has probiotics in it like yogurt (but we like to avoid dairy), sauerkraut, kimchi, kombucha (fermented green tea), and even pickles.

There are also "prebiotics," which are foods that nourish the bacteria. Prebiotics feed probiotics. Prebiotic foods include leeks, onions, asparagus, bananas, and garlic.

Repair:

We have removed the offending agents. We have added some good nutrients and possibly enzymes. You should already start feeling better. But now we must help heal the gut. This will take some time. We need certain foods and supplements to help with the healing. Certainly, a clean diet is already starting the work of healing, and the probiotics are fixing the microbiome but here I also like to add some supplemental support. I like to add collagen and amino acids, which also help to repair the gut (more details on these supplements in Chapter 6).

If you don't want to use supplements, eating bone broth is also a great way to repair the gut. Bone broth is sometimes called stock, it is *a broth made from boiling animal bones*. Chefs use stock as a base for soups, sauces, and gravies. But on its own, it is full of collagen and amino acids. People have been making bone broth since the beginning of humankind.

Bone broth is chock full of amino acids, collagen, gelatin, and minerals, which are great for healing leaky gut, improving dysbiosis, and helping your digestive tract in general, while also reducing inflammation.

IMPORTANT: *This is where the magic happens.*

As you go through this process notice how you feel. If possible, keep journal!

In our office, we use software to track all the symptoms but keeping a journal will do just as well

Pay attention to which things got better. What symptoms improved or disappeared altogether? Did the years of joint pain that you assumed was just arthritis go away? Did that ringing in the ears that you've been told will never go away suddenly disappear? Is the bloating gone? The years of constipation? How about your sleep. Are you suddenly sleeping through the night?

This is my favorite moment with my patients when they tell me (sometimes in tears) that they have never felt better. They can suddenly bend down to pick things up or suddenly have energy to exercise for the first time in years.

Pay attention to your symptoms

- Did your stomach discomfort lessen?
- Are you experiencing less bloating?
- Did your skin clear up?
- Are the headaches better?
- Did the ringing in your ears stop?
- Constipation/diarrhea improve?
- Are you sleeping through the night?
- Heart palpitations and sweating go away?

Pay attention to all of it. Even if you think it's not connected to your new diet, it probably is.

Once you start feeling better, you are officially a Game Changer. You have changed the course of your health destiny. Congratulations! You are amazing.

But there is another reason I want you to pay attention to the symptoms that improved. You need to know which things got better because we will use these symptoms to help us when it's time to Reintroduce some foods later.

The things that improved significantly with this diet are now considered your "tells." These are the things that will likely act up if you go back to your old habits. So, if a few months later if you are noticing that a symptom has returned, look at your diet and question what you have reintroduced.

Reintroduction:

At some point, you are going to want to bring back some of your favorites into your menu. This must be done methodically and carefully.

As I mentioned, be sure to pay attention to what symptoms improved or went away altogether. During this phase, they will be an important part of how to determine which food you can reintroduce later.

Stay on the diet as long as you can so that your gut can heal (at least a month but ideally longer like three to six months). Then, reintroduce new foods **SLOWLY** and **ONE AT A TIME**. Reintroduction needs to happen methodically. Each food you reintroduce should be eaten for a few meals in a row and then monitor your symptoms for at least three days after introduction. So, if you are adding chickpeas, add them at lunch or at dinner for two days in a row and see if anything changes. Remember it doesn't have to be just belly issues. Pay attention if your skin or joint issues return or if your brain fog returns. If nothing happened, you are clear to add this food back in to your life. If you have any symptoms, eliminate the food again, get back to baseline and try it again in a few weeks.

There are labs that can do this food sensitivity testing for you, but they are very expensive. This is a way that you can do it yourself and save money.

Start with the 4Rs by using the **REKNEW** diet in the Appendix. Consider adding intermittent fasting into your life (also in Appendix). If you are doing this, and if your symptoms are gone, your skin starts to clear up, and your hot flashes go away, guess what—you are done!

Stop here if you are feeling better after implementing the 4Rs and the **REKNEW DIET**. You can throw away this book. You are done. Or maybe give the book to someone you love so they can become the Game Changer in their life.

Let me say it again. Before you start spending your time and money on tests, start here. If you try the 4R protocol I've suggested thus far, and you still have persistent symptoms that are not being resolved, keep reading and only then start considering other possible diagnoses.

However, if you follow the protocol and eliminate all the inflammatory foods from your diet and you still don't feel good, or not good enough, that's when we go deep sea diving.

If you feel like you want to keep diving in the next few chapters, let's go!

CHAPTER 5:

TESTING FOR ADRENAL FATIGUE

YES, IT'S A REAL THING

Many of our clients come to us with one common complaint—they're exhausted. Many of them have trouble making it through the day without pumping themselves up with caffeine, power bars, and snacks. Some can't sleep at night or don't get deep restful sleep. Others are just feeling sluggish and don't know why.

They've done the bloodwork with their primary care providers, and some have seen specialists and have been tested for everything. But the tests all come back normal, so they come away with no answer, no diagnosis, and no treatment.

They are told that it is probably just stress and yes, the problems are likely related to stress, but there is far more to the picture than that. The concept that someone is just "stressed out" can give the wrong impression. Often, well-meaning people, including healthcare providers, put the responsibility back on the patient instead of getting to the root of the problem. The patient is told that "everything is fine," that they are not sick, and that there are no tests for the issues they're facing.

But there actually is a way to test for this.

When we test a person who is suffering from adrenal fatigue, we can see for the first time, in black and white, that what they're experiencing is quantifiable, measurable, and trackable. They are experiencing adrenal fatigue.

THE CORTISOL HORMONE:

To understand what is affecting adrenal fatigue, we must first talk about cortisol and the role it plays in your body.

Cortisol is what wakes you up in the morning. When things are working as they should, your cortisol level will be at its highest in the morning when you first wake up. Throughout the day, it will make a slow and steady decline as your body needs less and less of it. There will be no big dips or rises. It slowly fades down until the evening and should be lowest when it's time to go to sleep.

The graphic below represents the curve of cortisol in someone who is **NOT** suffering from adrenal fatigue.

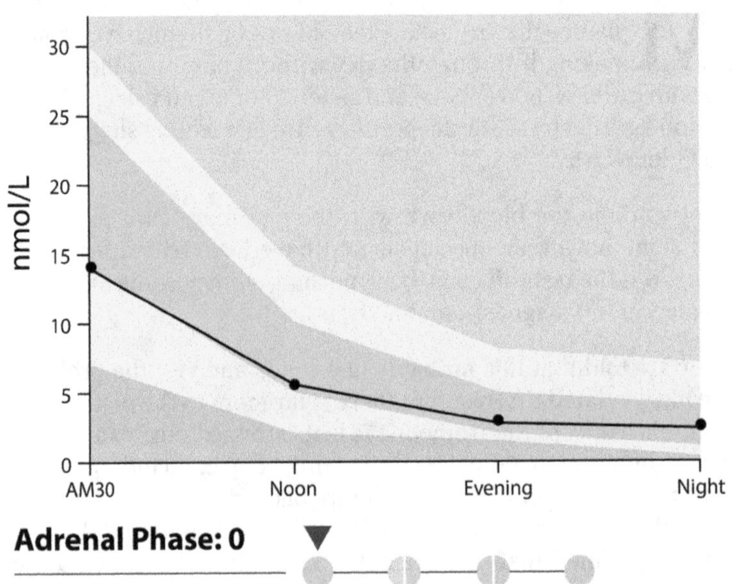

Cortisol Does More Than Just Wake You Up

You may have heard the expression "fight or flight." This refers to the way humans respond to danger and have for centuries. Our bodies are preset to respond to imminent danger. We either get set to fight when appropriate or take flight when the risk of harm is too great to handle. Cortisol is a part of that fight or flight response. Our bodies produce cortisol as needed to respond in appropriate measure to the danger at hand. If you were being chased by a lion, your cortisol would kick in so that you can figure out how to get out of its path. If you are walking down a dark street and think someone is following you, that energy you feel to start walking faster and be super alert is your fight or flight response. Part of that response is created by cortisol. In other words, cortisol is also your stress hormone. When you are stressed, your body will produce cortisol to get you through the stress.

Now, hopefully you are not being followed down the street every day or being chased by a lion, but you do have daily stress. We're bombarded throughout the day with phone calls, emails, and text messages that create constant stress. We have multiple responsibilities, picking up the kids, dealing with aging or sick parents, financial concerns, work deadlines, and more. All of it happening at the same time is stressful.

In addition to modern-day stressors, anyone who is living with chronic pain, chronic illness, or chronic fatigue is living with additional stressors. When our body perceives this, it will use our stored cortisol to meet the stress to deal with the deadline, get through the day, to help manage the chronic pain or fatigue.

If you were to use your cortisol in that manner occasionally, the curve we showed you in figure A would remain untouched. But if you consistently go to the cortisol bank to make withdrawals, that curve will lose its shape. And when that happens, it's called adrenal fatigue.

Think of it like an overdraft. Your body is taking cortisol withdrawals without making deposits. There are three levels of adrenal fatigue depending on how much reserve you have used.

THE THREE PHASES OF ADRENAL FATIGUE:

As we said, when we wake up, our body experiences a kind of arousal or excitement, so our adrenal glands produce the appropriate hormonal response, producing a spike in the production of cortisol. The normal production of cortisol becomes lower throughout the day, with no spikes or dips.

If this isn't the case, and the levels of cortisol production is abnormal, there are three phases of Adrenal Fatigue a person will likely fall into.

PHASE 1: They're overdrawn but by no means bankrupt. They may be experiencing some periods of tiredness, anxiety, maybe some brain fog. Some patients complain of a small weight gain. They might get a burst of energy around midday or evening, a spike of cortisol typically when at their busiest. That might be at lunch time, especially on a particularly stressful day, or, like many parents, at dinner when rushing around preparing food for the family. This is an inappropriate release of cortisol at the wrong time.

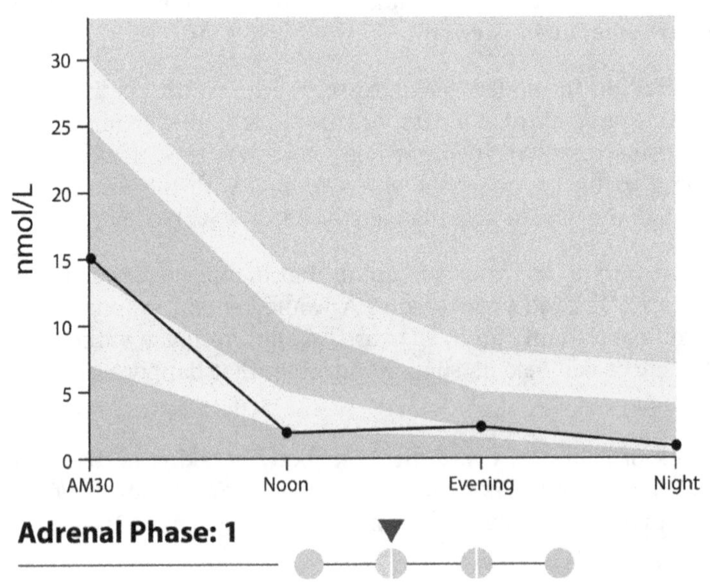

These events are noticeable but not debilitating. In fact, many people feel good in phase 1 because they feel energy during the time that they need it most and don't yet notice that they are depleting themselves in other parts of the day,

On the previous page is a typical curve of a person in phase 1 adrenal fatigue.

PHASE 2: The curve for a person in phase 2 of adrenal fatigue looks very similar to a normal curve but their cortisol level runs just under the green line and stays that much lower all through the day. (See graphic below) There are a couple of tells regarding your cortisol level in phase 2.

This person is not completely depleted. He or she will still have more energy in the morning then the rest of the day but feels tired and suboptimal throughout the day. They will reach for "pick-me-ups" like coffee, an energy drink, or some sugar to get the energy they are looking for. They may note increased anxiety and irritability, increased fatigue, and continuing weight gain. They are just a little tired all day. They may have a little trouble getting to sleep

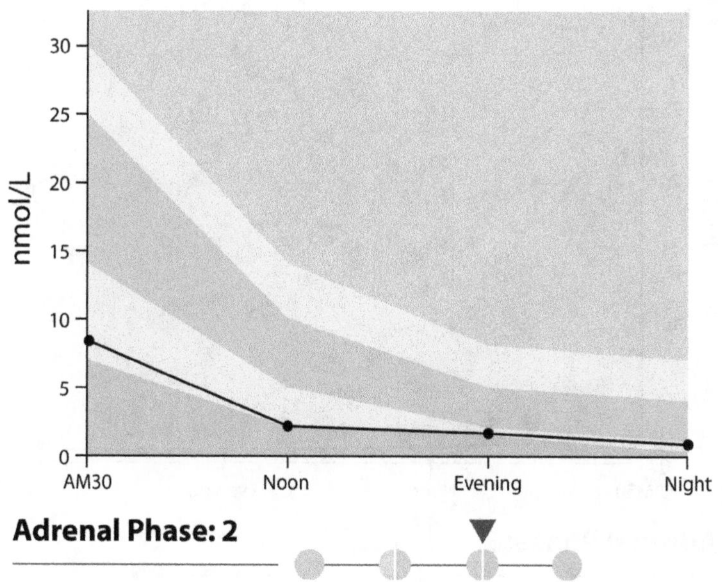

sometimes or getting good restful sleep. This adds to the fatigue and irritability during the day.

PHASE 3: When someone is in phase 3 adrenal fatigue, they lose the curve completely. There is no difference in the cortisol level from morning till night. This is the most severe stage. This patient is dragging all day.

If someone is in phase 3, they wake up exhausted and go to bed exhausted. All their measurements are low and, rather than having highs and lows, their curve is more like a flat line. They feel tired all the time. Their energy is depleted to the point where it feels like a herculean task to just get out of bed in the morning. No amount of sleep leaves this person feeling rested. They're moody, irritable, and depressed, can't concentrate, and have heavy brain fog. Their energy both day and night are equal. They're tired and sluggish all day and can't seem to accomplish much of anything because they are exhausted all the time.

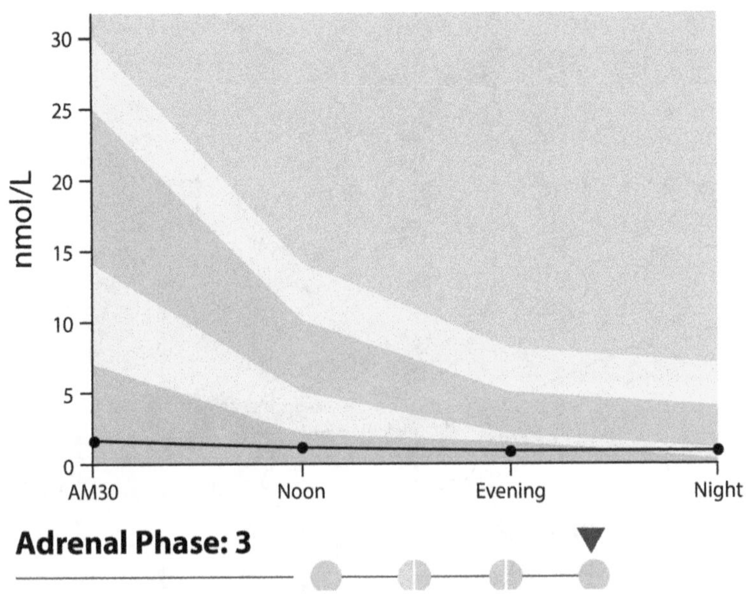

NOTE: People in phase 3 adrenal fatigue tend to feel exhausted after exercising to the point where they likely need a nap. Telling these patients to exercise might make them feel worse. We tell our phase 3 patients not to exercise until they have followed the protocols and begin to feel better.

These are some of the common symptoms of adrenal fatigue:

› You're exhausted a lot of the day
› It's hard to get up in the morning
› For some people, it's hard to fall asleep
› When you sleep, you don't feel rejuvenated
› You feel okay when you get up, but sometime during the day, you feel tired
› Your sex drive is decreased
› You find it hard to handle stress
› You might be recovering from a cold but feel dizzy when you try to stand up
› You suffer from mild depression
› You need to drink caffeinated beverages or snack a lot to get through the day
› You have brain fog
› You are getting less done than ever before

If any (or lots) of this sounds like what you're going through, you may be suffering from adrenal fatigue.

People suffering from adrenal fatigue, as the name suggests, lack energy. Their coping skills are declining. They get irritable more easily especially when hungry. No amount of rest changes the way they feel. They become frustrated with their situation especially when they seek medical advice and are told there is nothing wrong with them. They are likely burning the candle at both ends making it difficult to find the energy to handle any unexpected problem. For someone who has adrenal fatigue, even a small event like a flat tire can feel huge because they don't have the energy reserves to deal with it.

Having adrenal fatigue alone is exhausting but adding in a chronic issue or autoimmune coupled with adrenal fatigue makes it doubly exhausting.

How do I know if I have adrenal fatigue?

If you drink coffee every day to keep going or snack throughout the day, it may be more than just hunger. If you have a particular time during the day when you reach for a cookie or candy bar, for example, you know that 3 p.m. is cookie time, you might start to wonder if it's more than a love of Starbucks or Pepperidge Farm. It's more likely adrenal fatigue. Your adrenal glands can't keep up with the demand of the perceived fight or flight in your life, and your cortisol is depleted.

Meanwhile, your medical provider is telling you nothing is wrong, but your body is telling you something is, and it isn't in your head, it's in your physiology.

DO NOT SELF DIAGNOSE!

Just because these symptoms "sound" like you, it doesn't mean you have adrenal fatigue. These symptoms may be caused by other serious diseases. Make sure you go to your PCP first and be fully evaluated. If they suggest further testing, do that as well. Always rule out a pathology (disease) first. If everything comes back normal, and you're still exhausted, only then should you consider adrenal fatigue.

WHAT DOCTORS SAY ABOUT ADRENAL FATIGUE

P.S. DON'T BOTHER GOING TO YOUR ENDOCRINOLOGIST FOR THIS ISSUE.

Conventional medicine doesn't recognize adrenal fatigue. As far as adrenals go, most doctors will say there is no such thing as adrenal fatigue. Your adrenals are either working or they aren't, there is nothing in the middle. If the adrenals are overproducing cortisol, it is a disease called Cushing's Syndrome. If the adrenals are not producing enough, it is a disease called Addison's Disease. Both these diseases are serious and require immediate medical attention. We are not talking about these extremes here. We are talking about the people in the middle of the extremes. Traditional medicine recognizes these two extremes and nothing else in between.

This is true even in the testing. Your endocrinologist may ask for an early morning cortisol test and a 24-hour urine test. This gives information about your overall cortisol production but does not give any information about how you are doing throughout the day.

I love and respect endocrinologists. When it comes to adrenal fatigue, we are looking for different things. What they are looking for are diagnoses that are critical and important and can save lives. What I am looking for are answers to why you are not feeling optimal throughout the day.

Below is an example of a person we worked with who was in phase 3 adrenal fatigue.

A CASE STUDY: PATIENT JL

JL was a 55-year-old female who came to us because she just didn't "feel like herself." The patient stated that she felt tired all the time, her stomach never felt "right," and she had vague muscle aches. She told us that she used to be an early riser, but now found it very difficult to wake up in the morning and that she had a hard time falling asleep.

She described her muscle aches as being "all over," and not so much presenting as pain but rather like a heaviness she felt all over her body, most predominantly in her upper back and shoulders.

Regarding her stomach issues, she told us she always felt very bloated even after small meals, and she had been feeling this way for about 18 months. She had seen her Primary Care Physician (PCP) for her symptoms several times who told her that everything was okay and suggested that perhaps it was just menopause (which had already occurred at age 53). JL denied having any other medical history, and her only surgery was a tonsillectomy at age 9. She had gone to her gastroenterology doctor for an endoscopy and a colonoscopy. In addition, she had already seen a neurologist and rheumatologist to discuss her muscle heaviness.

Like most people, she was convinced that something must be wrong with her thyroid, which would explain her fatigue. She asked her primary care physician to run a thyroid test which came back normal, but she remained convinced that it was her thyroid.

She filled out our comprehensive questionnaire and claimed her fatigue level was a 4 out of 4.

We ran a full panel on her and found her thyroid having no issues, but her saliva showed phase 3 adrenal fatigue, which is the most severe stage of adrenal fatigue. This was in keeping with the symptoms she was experiencing: extreme exhaustion, stomach issues, low energy, moodiness, and depression as well as sleep issues.

How we addressed her problems

We began by cleaning up her diet. We started with diet because (as you should know by now) we always start with the gut. We start by removing the toxins but in her case, we also put her on supplements for adrenal support, which she took every morning and at noon.

Early results

Within one month, she was able to get up in the morning. By the end of the second month, she was able to slowly start exercising and stated that for the first time in years, she wasn't depleted after working out.

By month four, she was on a full exercise program and by this point, the exercise was invigorating and didn't leave her wiped out.

WHEN IS TESTING NEEDED?

You don't necessarily have to test for adrenal fatigue. If you have access to a functional medicine provider, or if you can come to us for help, great. But if you can't do so and are feeling these symptoms, the first thing you do is go to your PCP and let them rule out any underlying causes. You want to be certain there is nothing more serious at play, and it's important that you eliminate any serious illnesses or issues they can test for.

Once your primary provider has run all the tests and you come away with no diagnosis and you're not anemic, your thyroid is functioning properly, you have no chronic issues or illnesses, and in fact, "you're fine," you can assume that you have adrenal fatigue. Start with the protocols in this book and see if you feel better. You have nothing to lose by making these healthy choices.

If there is a functional medicine facility within your reach, it's great to get tested, to know what you are dealing with and to feel validated about what you are experiencing. If you choose to get tested, there is a saliva test that any functional medical provider can do. I recommend at a least a "four-point test." The test measures your cortisol at 4 different times throughout the day. We do a 4-point test starting with when the patient first gets up, then a second, right at lunch. The third time is early evening around dinner time, and the fourth time is right before going to sleep.

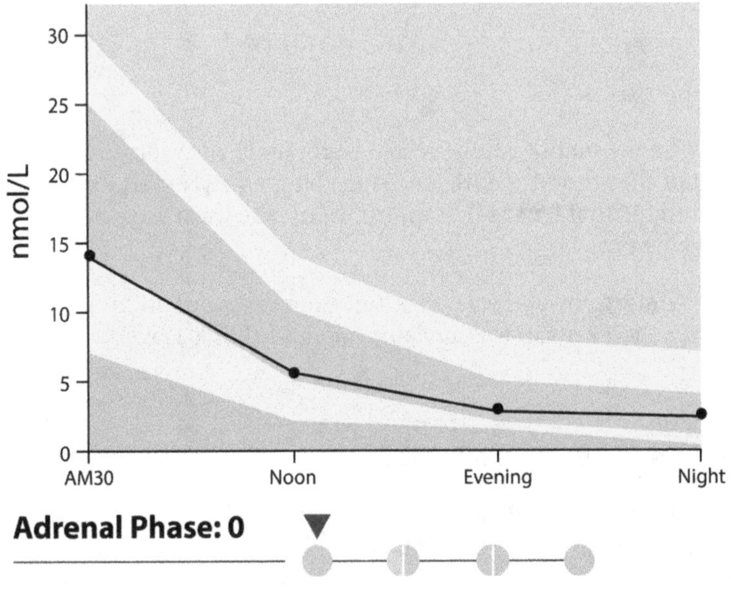

As we said above, this is the perfect curve, high in the morning, gradually declining during the day.

Remember, no matter what phase of adrenal fatigue you're in, this did not happen overnight. It took some time to get to this place, and it will take some time to repair it. There are NO quick fixes. It may take several months and certainly requires an openness to change, but this can absolutely be reversed, and you can absolutely start feeling better again.

Okay, I have adrenal fatigue but how do I fix it?

SOME OF THE THINGS WE ADDRESS TO FIX OR REDUCE ADRENAL FATIGUE:

Diet:

Since this is an issue of over stressing the system, we must remove the stress. When I say remove the stress, I don't mean we have to meditate every day (although that is a good thing to do). Of course, I want you to find way to manage your stress. However, this takes time and practice. There is something you can do immediately to reduce your stress level and that is to change your diet.

The number one stressor for most people is how they eat. This is why we always start with the diet. Considering the amount of toxins we put in our body, including the processed food, chemicals, and sugar we consume, we must realize that we are asking our bodies to work hard. If we start by changing our diet, adding good, whole foods and reducing the toxins, we will reduce our stress by a great deal. Start with the 4Rs and the ReKnew Diet.

Exercise:

Believe it or not, over exercising is also a stressor, particularly for people in phase 2 or 3 of adrenal fatigue. The body doesn't know that you are running on a treadmill by choice. It thinks you are being chased. When you exercise, you are using your cortisol. If you are already in adrenal fatigue and using your reserves, overexercising may be creating more stress for your body. It's important to find a balance of exercise that leaves you feeling invigorated and not depleted.

If you do want to exercise, it's best to do so in the morning when the cortisol levels in your body are high. If you choose to exercise in the evening, you may notice that it is hard for you to wind down for sleep in the evening and that is because the exercise increased your cortisol levels.

If your schedule only allows you to exercise in the evening, that's okay, we always meet the patient where they are. It's just important to know that this may affect your sleep later in the evening.

Regular physical activity can increase the production of hormones that:

- make you feel happier
- help you sleep better
- help you lose weight and keep it off
- improve your skin's appearance

Just don't overdo it! If you feel that you must take a nap after you exercise, this is an indication that you have adrenal fatigue, so instead of pushing yourself, work on repairing your adrenals first. You will see that you will get your energy back and feel like exercising again.

Sleep:

Sleep is critical for reducing stress. Not sleeping enough or not getting restful sleep is a huge stressor. Getting good sleep has a variety of benefits includes helping curb weight gain, improving memory, and boosting your immune system. You know what happens when you don't sleep for a night or sleep badly. You find yourself slogging through your daily activities, and everything hurts more. You go through the day, moody and irritable. Now multiply that by every night, and you have constant physical stress.

Everyone wants to sleep, but for some of you, this may prove to be a hard task. Some of you have difficulty falling asleep, and others can fall asleep but toss and turn at night. Often, this has to do with your diet during the day. Cleaning up your diet will have a huge impact on your sleep.

We forget sometimes that it's all connected. What you do during the day will affect your sleep. Look at how many stimulants like caffeine and sugar you consume, especially after lunch; this will affect your sleep. What you eat for dinner is also critical. Having a heavy meal with a glass of wine may make you feel sleepy, but it will certainly disrupt your sleep as your body works to break it all down during the night. **IT'S ALL CONNECTED.**

Relaxation Techniques:

So, if you have changed your diet, created a good exercise regimen that is not overdoing it, and you are getting good restful sleep, consider adding relaxation techniques. Meditation and deep breathing can reduce stress. A walk in the fresh air, some light yoga, and/or a stress-free hobby that takes your mind off things can also be helpful.

It can start as simply as learning to embrace gratitude. Gratitude is not an action; it is a mindset that starts by becoming aware of and thankful for the good things in your life. It can be noticing a beautiful sunset, feeling loved by a friend, or petting your dog. When you focus on the good things, even when times are tough, it helps to shift your perspective and improve your mood. All of these are ways to reduce stress.

I didn't do a deep discussion of relaxation techniques in this book. There are plenty of books that you can read about how to relax. You already know that finding a way to reduce stress is important, and I agree with that, however, if your diet consists of McDonalds and Coke, all the meditation in the world won't counterbalance that.

This is why I always start by removing one of the biggest stressors to the body which is the Standard American Diet. I said it was sad before. It still is.

Supplements and Vitamins:

There are also certain supplements and vitamins that can help support the adrenal system. We will discuss them further in Chapter 6.

What I want you to get from this chapter is that your fatigue can be explained. Your symptoms are not in your head. If you have adrenal fatigue, it can be managed, and the symptoms can be reduced or even eliminated. The most important element in managing adrenal fatigue is YOU. Only you can make the changes necessary to feel better. You must be the game changer in your life.

CHAPTER 6:

WHAT ABOUT SUPPLEMENTS?

There are literally thousands of supplements available in the marketplace, and there are misconceptions about the way supplements work to support a healthy body. I'm a firm believer in taking supplements when appropriate. I take them, and I encourage my patients to take them.

However, supplements do not replace food. You still must "eat the rainbow." If you don't like eating green leafy vegetables, I'm here to tell you, "Get over it!" You need them. Your body needs the nutrients that you're going to get from good whole foods. Supplements are what I call "part of this complete breakfast" (do you remember that from cereal commercials?). Get rid of the Standard American Diet, add good nutritious food and then top it off with some top-notch supplements.

This chapter is certainly not a comprehensive guide to supplements. That would require a very, very, very big (and boring) book. I am going to focus on the ones we use most in my practice. I will start with the four supplements that I encourage just about everyone to take, and then I will go over some supplements that we recommend depending on the patient's circumstances.

Let's start with the four supplements that I recommend to almost all my patients: **MULTIVITAMIN, VITAMIN D, NAC, AND OMEGA 3**

MULTIVITAMINS:

If we eat a very well-balanced, whole-foods diet, we can get lots of the nutrients we need each day from our food, particularly fruits and vegetables. The truth is, most of us are unable to get all the nutrients we need just from eating. To counterbalance that fact, many people take a multivitamin.

Multivitamins contain the different vitamins and minerals that are considered essential for balanced nutritional health. There is no standard for what makes up a multivitamin, and they can come in capsules, tablets, chewable, and even liquid form. Their composition can vary quite a lot from brand to brand, so it's important to know what makes up a quality multivitamin. We have one we consider the best to recommend for our patients.

Think of a multivitamin as a kind of insurance policy for your body. If you don't get all the vitamins and minerals your body needs from the food you eat, your multivitamin fills in the gaps.

Multivitamins can help in many ways:

- Promote heart health
- Enhance healthy aging by giving us much-needed nutrients
- Boost your immune system and energy levels
- Decrease the feelings of anxiety and stress
- Reduce the risk of diseases, especially cancer
- Support healthy eyes, hair, and skin
- Give us a feeling of general well-being

It's imperative to get a good quality multivitamin. On the next page is a chart listing the ingredients of the multivitamin we recommend. Be sure you not only have the list of these vitamins in your vitamin bottle but also the dosages. (We don't have any financial connections to this company, it's just a multivitamin we like to use in the practice.)

O.N.E.™ Multivitamin

Supplement Facts	
Amount Per Serving	
Each (size 00) vegetarian capsule contains:	
Vitamin A (as vitamin A acetate and 73% beta carotene)	1,125 mcg
Vitamin C (as ascorbic acid)	180 mg
Vitamin D (as cholecalciferol) (D_3)	50 mcg (2,000 IU)
Vitamin E (as d-alpha tocopherol succinate)	20 mg
Thiamin (as thiamin HCl) (B_1)	3 mg
Riboflavin (as vitamin B_2 and 43% riboflavin 5' phosphate (activated B_2))	3 mg
Niacin (as niacinamide)	20 mg
Vitamin B_6 (as pyridoxine HCl and 38% pyridoxal 5' phosphate (activated B_6))	4 mg
< Folate (as Metafolin®, L-5-MTHF)	667 mcg DFE (400 mcg L-5-MTHF)
Vitamin B_{12} (as methylcobalamin)	500 mcg
Biotin	300 mcg
Pantothenic acid (as calcium pantothenate) (B_5)	10 mg
Choline (as choline bitartrate)	25 mg
Iodine (as potassium iodide)	150 mcg
Zinc (as zinc citrate)	25 mg
Selenium (as selenomethionine)	70 mcg
Manganese (as manganese citrate)	2 mg
Chromium (as chromium polynicotinate)	200 mcg
Molybdenum (as TRAACS® molybdenum glycinate chelate)	75 mcg
Boron (as boron glycinate)	1 mg
Inositol	25 mg
Coenzyme Q_{10} (as CoQ_{10} and as 18% from MicroActive® CoQ_{10}-cyclodextrin complex	50 mg
Alpha lipoic acid	50 mg
FloraGLO® lutein	3 mg
Zeaxanthin	500 mcg
Lycopene	500 mcg
Other ingredients: vegetarian capsule (cellulose, water), hypoallergenic plant fiber (cellulose), ascorbyl palmitate, potato starch	

VITAMIN D: IT'S NOT JUST FOR YOUR BONES

Most of us know that Vitamin D plays an essential role in protecting our bones and teeth, but Vitamin D has also been found useful in preventing and treating skin issues, musculoskeletal issues, neuromuscular function, immune function, and even affects insulin levels. Also, laboratory studies have shown that Vitamin D can reduce cancer cell growth, help control infections, and reduce inflammation. Many of the body's organs and tissues have receptors for Vitamin D, which suggest important roles beyond bone health, and scientists are actively investigating other possible functions.

Vitamin D can help with the:

- absorption of calcium
- protection of our bones, teeth, and muscle
- function of our immune system
- health of our lungs and hearts

› regulation of insulin levels to support the management of diabetes

Aside from fatty fish, there aren't many foods that are rich in Vitamin D, so most diets do not give us enough intake of Vitamin D.

There was a time when humans had enough exposure to sunlight, which is another way in which we can make Vitamin D. Unfortunately, most of us don't get enough sunlight, which is why supplementing is the best solution. Adequate and sensible sun exposure, as a source of Vitamin D, is usually best when there is an exposure of the arms and legs for about 5 to 30 minutes, twice a week. This may be enough, but it really depends on the time of day, season, latitude, and age of patient.

As a supplement, the recommended dosage depends on your starting point. The goal is to be above 30 Nanograms/ml but never above 100 Nanograms/ml. If you have a true Vitamin D deficiency, you will likely need a higher dose of about 5,000 IU/daily for about eight weeks followed by a maintenance dose of 1,500-2,000 IU/daily.

It is important to not overdo it with vitamin D because it is fat soluble, which means it is stored in the body and can accumulate in your tissues and become toxic. So, have your levels checked before you start taking it as a supplement.

N-ACETYL CYSTEINE (NAC):

NAC breaks down into an antioxidant called glutathione, which is magical. (Well, not really magic but it is awesome.) Let's take a moment to understand what it is and why we need it. It starts with something called oxidative stress.

There is a war in your body between free radicals (the bad guys) vs. antioxidants (the good guys). Free radicals have an extra wild electron that can cause damage. An antioxidant can calm that free radical down by giving it an electron. When there is an imbalance between these two, it can cause oxidative stress.

This oxidative stress can damage the body on a cellular level. It can damage proteins, lipids, and DNA which, over time, can lead to diseases. A few examples include heart disease, Parkinson's disease, and various inflammatory conditions.

As I said, antioxidants combat these free radicals. One of the body's most powerful antioxidants is glutathione because it provides antioxidation protection in the tissues and respiratory tract. In short, glutathione helps prevent damage in your body. You see, I told you it's magical.

We do have our own natural supply of glutathione, which is made by our liver. But production of this can be slowed or halted by poor diet, aging, trauma, infections and/or stress. To help boost production of glutathione, we recommend taking NAC.

Some of the benefits of the NAC supplement:

- Essential for making the powerful antioxidant glutathione
- Repairs damaged liver cells and helps detoxify the liver
- Helps reduce inflammation
- Slows the loss of cognitive ability for people with Alzheimer's disease
- Helps relieve symptoms of respiratory conditions
- May decrease inflammation in fat cells, stabilize blood sugar, and improve insulin resistance
- May lower the risk of heart disease because it may reduce oxidative damage to the tissues in your heart and helps improve blood flow
- May alleviate the symptoms of some psychiatric disorders by regulating glutamate levels in your brain and may also reduce the tendency to addictive behaviors.
- Helps with your body's detoxification process the side effects caused by taking certain drugs and the effects of environmental toxins.

There is no recommended daily allowance because it is not an essential nutrient. Most frequently used oral dosages of NAC in clinical trials have been 600-1,200 mg/day, usually administered in three divided doses/day.

OMEGA 3

Omega 3 fatty acids are a family of essential fatty acids that play very important roles in the body by providing several health benefits. When something is essential, that means your body can't produce so you must ingest it. Omega 3 fatty acids are super important and are made up of three fatty acids called ALA, EPA, and DHA. Foods that are high in omega-3 fatty acids include fatty fish, fish oils, flax seeds, chia seeds, flaxseed oil, and walnuts.

ALA

Alpha-linolenic acid (ALA) is the most common of the omega-3 fatty acids found in most people's diet. ALA is essential because the body cannot make it, which means we must get it in our diet or in a supplement.

Benefits of ALA:

- helps decrease the risk of heart disease
- assists in maintaining a normal heart rhythm.
- may help patients suffering with heart-related diseases such as high blood pressure and hardening of the arteries, and it may help reduce blood clots
- it is the fatty acid used for the synthesis of EPA and DHA

We can get ALA from foods like flaxseeds, flaxseed oil, chia seeds, walnuts, hemp seeds, and soybeans.

EPA

Eicosatetraenoic acid (EPA) is mostly found in animal products, such as fatty fish and fish oil. However, some microalgae also contain EPA. It has several functions in your body and has an anti-inflammatory effect.

Benefits of EPA:

- prevents the blood from clotting easily
- reduces triglyceride levels in the blood
- lowers risk of cardiovascular disease.
- slows the progression of rheumatoid arthritis
- helps lower chronic pain and inflammation

DHA

One of the most important omega-3 fatty acids in your body is Docosahexaenoic acid (DHA). It's a key structural component of your brain, the retina of your eyes, and numerous other body parts. We mainly get DHA from fatty fish and fish oil, but we can get a great deal of it from dairy products and meat (preferably from animals that are grass fed). DHA also plays a role in the development of the central nervous system and the retina.

We suggest to anyone who is vegan or even vegetarian that they take microalgae supplements for DHA because they will often be lacking this nutrient.

Benefits of DHA:

- helps with depression, mood swings, and bipolar symptoms
- assists with brain-based disorders such as cognitive decline
- contributes to improved memory function in older adults
- helps manage inflammation
- offers blood vessel and blood-clotting support

Balancing Omegas in the Body

There are three major families of fatty acids in the diet—Omega 3, Omega 6, and Omega 9. All three are important to the body, but it is important to have a good ratio of them. Unfortunately, the Standard American Diet creates an imbalance between Omega 3 and Omega 6, meaning that most Americans will have a much higher amount of omega 6 in their bodies than Omega 3. Omega

6, at high levels, is pro inflammatory, so it is important to change that ratio. This explains why taking Omega 3 as a supplement or eating sources of Omega 3 are important.

So, not only are we taking Omega 3 for its health benefits, but we are also taking it to improve the balance between Omega 3 and the relative deficiency in Omega 3 in the western diet, which explains why supplementation is so beneficial. Dosages vary between 1 to 12g per day for fish oil. You can also get vegan sources of Omega 3 in flaxseed and there the recommended dosage for a supplement is 5 to 30 ml/day.

The rest of the supplements in this chapter are patient specific. Depending on the individual patient needs, we may recommend these other supplements:

TURMERIC

We often recommend turmeric for reduction of pain caused by inflammation.

Turmeric is a common household spice whose main active ingredient is something called curcumin. That is what gives it the yellow color you might recognize. This comes from a plant related to ginger and is grown in many Asian countries. It has anti-inflammatory benefits. Many people don't realize that this spice—Curcumin—is particularly helpful in pain reduction and ease of movement for people with osteoarthritis or arthritis because of its anti-inflammatory qualities. There are even studies that suggest taking turmeric three times a day is equal to taking 1,200 milligrams of ibuprofen per day! Part of the plant can be dried and is used to make as a supplement in capsules or tablets as well as in teas and powders.

There has been a lot of research on the benefits of curcumin:

- reduces cholesterol and triglyceride levels in the body
- lessens some of the symptoms of rheumatoid arthritis such as joint swelling and stiffness.

- reduces the symptoms of Crohn's disease
- helps with depression
- reduces the symptoms of irritable bowel syndrome (IBS)

DOSAGE: Turmeric is considered generally safe if you are taking less than 8 grams a day, although that varies depending on a person's particular needs and health conditions. For some people, turmeric can cause stomach upset. If you experience this, please stop taking the supplement or reduce your dosage.

FOR PATIENTS WHO NEED METHYLATION SUPPORT AND PATIENTS WITH MTHFR MUTATIONS.

SERIOUS NERD ALERT

To understand methylation, we first must talk about methyl groups. A methyl group consists of one carbon and three hydrogens. When a methyl group attaches to a molecule, or is passed from one molecule to another, it's a way of telling the molecule to start doing its work.

In general, methyl groups and methylation are amazing because it happens all over the body all the time. When methylation is going well, the process helps:

- repair your DNA
- regulate your hormones
- produce energy
- protect against cancer
- support detoxification
- keep your immune system healthy
- support the protective coating along your nerves
- strengthen the nervous system
- and on and on ...

But some people have a genetic defect in the enzyme that regulates methylation. This genetic defect is in the gene called MTHFR. People who have this mutation have a hard time with methylation.

Symptoms of undermethylation can include:

- anxiety
- depression
- insomnia
- IBD
- allergies
- headaches
- GI issues
- muscle pain

When people have a hard time methylating, their B2, B12 and folic acid are not bioavailable, which, simply put, means that they are not active. There is a gene called MTHFR, which is responsible for methylation in every cell of your body. Some people have a mutation in that gene. MTHFR mutation can cause people to not produce enough methyl groups.

We can't talk about MTHFR without also mentioning homocysteine, which is something that we test for with all our patients. Here is just one way homocysteine MTHFR affects your body, but it is important to discuss.

HYPERHOMOCYSTEINEMIA

Homocysteine is an amino acid that is not found in food. It is made by a process called "demethylation." Basically, this means taking away a "methyl" group from the molecule. It's important to have the right amount of homocysteine in the body. Too much of it is not good, and when this happens, it is called Hyperhomocysteinemia.

High homocysteine can affect:

- coronary artery disease
- diabetes
- GI disorders like IBD and colon cancer
- impairment of bone health

› and it can contribute to Alzheimer's, Parkinson's, and mood disorders

The most effective way to bring these levels down is to help convert the homocysteine into a different amino acid called methionine. The way to do that is by "methylating" the homocysteine, which means adding a "methyl group" to it. But, as I mentioned, some people with a MTHFR mutation have a hard time methylating. These groups of people need extra support with supplements that have methyl groups already in them. We give them a supplement full of methylated B vitamins.

A neat trick that the body does is that when homocysteine is successfully lowered, that process also increases glutathione (see above for more info on glutathione). So, when we take these vitamins, we get a two-for-one special.

If you have a hard time methylating, it can affect so much of your health. The solution is simple; take a supplement full of methylated B vitamins.

DOSAGE: The methyl supplements we recommend for our patients are 1,000 mcg/pill and the recommended dose is 3,000mcg.

For patients with low vitamin A:

Though Vitamin A is often considered a singular nutrient, it's really the name for a group of fat-soluble compounds, including retinol, retinal, and retinyl esters.

There are two forms of Vitamin A found in food, preformed and provitamin.

Preformed vitamin A—retinol and retinyl esters—are found in animal products, such as dairy, liver, and fish. Provitamin A carotenoids are found in plant foods like fruits, vegetables, and oils. To use them, your body must convert both forms of Vitamin A to retinal and retinoic acid, the active forms of the vitamin.

Most of the Vitamin A in your body is kept in your liver in the form of retinyl esters. These esters are then broken down and then enter your bloodstream, at which point your body can use it. Because Vitamin A is fat soluble, it's stored in body tissue for later use.

Vitamin A plays a role in:

- maintaining tissues in the skin, GI, respiratory tract, nose, and urinary tract
- maintaining your body's natural defenses by supporting immune function, it also supports the growth and distribution of T-cells, a type of white blood cell that protects your body from infection
- visual functions such as color vision and low-light vision. It also helps protect and maintain the cornea, the outermost layer of your eye and the conjunctiva, a thin membrane that covers the surface of your eye and inside of your eyelids
- immune function
- serving as an antioxidant
- and studies show a decreased risk of certain types of cancer, including Hodgkin's lymphoma, cervical, lung and bladder cancer.

Having a deficiency in Vitamin A can increase your susceptibility to infections and delay your recovery when you get sick because a Vitamin A deficiency decreases our immunity.

Vitamin A, like vitamin D is a fat-soluble vitamin that is stored in your body (just like Vitamin D). Because your body stores it, dosing is important, meaning you can have too much Vitamin A. Too much Vitamin A consumption can lead to toxic levels. It must be taking in moderation, or it can cause serious side effects.

Best dosage varies between 5 to 25/a day depending on the level needed or if you are experiencing night blindness.

FOR PATIENTS WITH GUT ISSUES: PROBIOTICS

When we are talking about good gut health, we often need to replace good bacteria to restore balance. This means we need probiotics. (See Chapter 4) You can get probiotics from certain foods like yogurt, kimchee, and even pickles, but you can also get what you need by simply taking a probiotic supplement.

Probiotics consist of good live bacteria like those that live naturally your body. As we've said before, we always have both good and bad bacteria in our bodies, and that's a good thing. But when the system gets out of balance, we wind up with more bad bacteria than good. That's when we need to add more of the good to the balance sheet. The good bacteria we add, in the form of probiotics, helps eliminate the extra bad bacteria and restore balance to our systems. Probiotics are bacteria that have beneficial effects on human health. They have been linked to helping various GI issues, including colic, constipation, IBS, H pylori, and other conditions.

Be careful though. Some people may not be ready to start on probiotics right away. They may need to undergo a few weeks of eliminating certain foods from their diet before starting on probiotics. I usually start my patient on probiotics only after a month of a clean diet. Remember the 4 R's. We remove first; reinoculation starts later. If we start probiotics too soon, it can lead to a worsening of symptoms.

There are a wide range of probiotic strains. The probiotics that we recommend have Saccharomyces boulardi, Lactobacillus acidophilus, and Bacillus coagulants as well as Arabinogalactan in them.

Saccharomyces Boulardii

This is often used to prevent the growth of harmful bacteria in the stomach and intestines. S. boulardii has demonstrated to be effective on some inflammatory gastrointestinal diseases.

DDS -1 Lactobacillus Acidophilus

This probiotic bacteria is found naturally in the gut and other parts of the human body. It helps the digestive system break sugar down into lactic acid. Like many other probiotics, you can get it in yogurt and fermented foods. Consuming L. acidophilus helps put good bacteria into the intestines.

Bacillus Coagulans

This probiotic is a beneficial bacteria and it can help boost the immune system and is also thought to help treat some of the symptoms of irritable bowel syndrome (IBS) and other inflammatory bowel and stomach diseases.

Arabino Galactan

Arabinogalactan is the main ingredient in plant gums like gum arabic. It's a natural compound found in many plants. It may offer help with boosting the immune system and lowering cholesterol levels. Other health benefits include preventing common colds, improving vaccine response, and there is evidence that it can help with diabetes.

Probiotic dosage is written as "CFU" or colony forming units. This estimates the number of live microbes capable of forming colonies in laboratory testing. CFU is determined in the laboratory because it tells you the viability of the bacteria before they're exposed to in the GI tract.

We recommend a product with 30 billion CFU. A daily dose of 10-20 billion CFU is advisable for individuals seeking everyday immune and digestive support.

FOR PATIENTS WITH ADRENAL FATIGUE, we recommend adaptogens and glandulars.

ADAPTOGENS:

Adaptogens are certain herbs or mushrooms that can help with stress and adrenal fatigue. These herbs help our bodies in reacting to or recovering from both short- and long-term physical or mental stress. Research shows adaptogens can fight fatigue, enhance mental performance, improve depression and anxiety, and they help you feel amazing and not just dragging through the day.

We are designed to be "live wires" in the morning and to cool down and rest by early evening, so we want to take adaptogens earlier in the day before 3 p.m. to align with the body's natural rhythms.

There are several different kinds of adaptogens; the product we use has the following adaptogens in it.

Here are some adaptogens and how they can help:

- Ashwagandha can reduce stress and anxiety
- Asian Ginseng Extract to improve physical stamina, concentration, and memory
- Holy Basil Extract is known to reduce stress
- Rhodiola Extract staves off physical and mental fatigue
- Eleuthero Extract improves focus
- Pantetheine can downregulate hypersecretion of cortisol secondary to high-stress conditions
- Boerhavia Extract significantly decreases stress induced, elevated levels of cortisol
- Betaine HCl Peptidase are added because when we are stressed, as a rule, this results in the body allocating its resources away from digestion and stomach acid production and into the physical stress response through cortisol production
- Vitamin C helps reduce both the physical and psychological effects of stress

GLANDULAR THERAPY

This refers to the use of animal tissues to try to enhance the function of, or mimic the effect of, the corresponding human tissue. Essentially, these animal tissues are dried and ground up for use in supplements and medications. Typically, glandular tissues come from cows, sheep, and pigs.

Adrenal extract (oral) is used for:

- low adrenal function

- fatigue
- stress
- impaired resistance to illness
- severe allergies
- asthma
- eczema
- psoriasis
- rheumatoid arthritis
- and other inflammatory conditions

The supplement that we use in our office also has, in addition to the glandulars, high-potency vitamins B1, B5, B6, and C. Like adaptogens, we recommend taking these before 3 p.m. to increase energy in line with our body's natural rhythm.

NOTE: For people who have progressed to Stage 3 adrenal fatigue, we might consider a low dose of Cortef, which is a medicine containing hydrocortisone that can be used as a cortisol replacement in people with adrenal insufficiency when the adrenal glands are not producing enough natural steroids. For this population, sometimes supplements alone are not enough.

FOR PATIENTS WHO ARE ANEMIC: IRON

Iron is a mineral that's necessary for life. Iron plays a key role in the making of red blood cells, which carry oxygen. You can get iron from food and from supplements. If you don't have enough iron, you may develop anemia, a low level of red blood cells. However, most people in the U.S. get their iron from food.

For our patients who are anemic or iron deficient, we like a product called HemeVite™, which is "intended to support hemoglobin synthesis by providing ferrous fumarate, a good source of iron, which is part of hemoglobin and essential for the delivery of oxygen to the tissues. Iron is also needed for mitochondrial support and creating thyroid hormones. This formulation also includes Vitamin C, which helps the body absorb the consuming of HemeVite™ and calcium (dairy) at the same time." (https://apexenergetics.com/hemevite)

Side effects include constipation, so it is usually better to increase slowly and see how it affects your digestion. It is possible to overdose on iron because you can get iron toxicity, so don't overdo it.

Common dose is 50-60 mg twice a day with food. This usually causes GI issues, so sometimes 30mg is handled better. Taking it with Vitamin C is handled better. Usually, iron improves within 6-12 weeks but for some people, it may take longer.

FOR PATIENTS WHO STRUGGLE WITH SLEEP: MELATONIN

Melatonin is a hormone made from tryptophan, which your brain produces in response to darkness. It helps with the timing of your circadian rhythms (your 24-hour internal clock) and enhances sleep. Your melatonin level starts to rise when it's dark outside, signaling to your body that it's time to sleep. It then decreases in the morning when it's light outside to promote wakefulness. Being exposed to light at night (which many of us are with phones and electronics) can block melatonin production and disrupt our sleep. Melatonin lets your body know it's time to sleep. It does not "knock you out." It's just a signal for your body that it's time to get ready for bed.

DOSING: Less is more. Take 1 to 3 milligrams two hours before bedtime, and if melatonin for sleep isn't helping after a week or two, stop using it. There are a lot of drug interactions with melatonin, so be sure to discuss this with your provider before taking it.

FOR PATIENTS WITH ELEVATED CHOLESTEROL: RED YEAST RICE & CO Q10

This is fermented rice produced by growing red yeast on white rice. It produces a substance called monacolins, which are very similar to statin (cholesterol-lowering drugs). It slows down the production of cholesterol. In clinical trials, it has reduced serum total cholesterol and LDL levels. Side effects are uncommon, unlike with a statin.

Red yeast rice may depreciate an important nutrient called Coenzyme q10, so patients should also take coq10 at about 30mg per day with this. The supplement that we like to use has both ingredients in it. The dose for red yeast rice should be 1,200-2,400 mg daily. For everyone who is taking red yeast rice, we recommend that they also take Coq 10. Your cells use CoQ10 for growth and maintenance. We need CoQ10 for so many things in our body, yet the levels of CoQ10 in your body decrease as you age. CoQ10 levels have also been found to be lower in people with certain conditions, such as heart disease, and in those who are taking cholesterol-lowering drugs or statins.

Red Yeast Rice

This is fermented rice produced by growing red yeast on white rice. It produces a substance called monacolin, which is very similar to statins (cholesterol-lowering drugs). In fact, this is so similar to the medication that the FDA likes to regulate how much is allowed in a supplement. It slows down the production of cholesterol. In clinical trials, it reduced serum total cholesterol and LDL levels. Side effects are uncommon, unlike statins. Additionally red yeast rice is also used to promote heart health and reduce inflammation.

It is important to get a high-quality supplement because red yeast rice needs to be carefully cultivated. If not carefully made, it can contain a byproduct called citrinin which can be harmful.

Dosing:

Dosing ranges from 1200-2400 daily divided into 2-3 doses.

What CoQ10 helps with:

› **HEART CONDITIONS.** CoQ10 has been shown to improve symptoms of congestive heart failure. CoQ10 might help reduce blood pressure. Some research also suggests that when combined with other nutrients, CoQ10 might aid recovery in people who've had bypass and heart valve surgery.

- **DIABETES.** Although more studies are needed, some research suggests that CoQ10 may help reduce low-density lipoprotein (LDL) cholesterol and total cholesterol levels in people with diabetes, lowering their risk of heart disease.
- **STATIN-INDUCED MYOPATHY.** Some research suggests that CoQ10 might ease the muscle weakness and pain sometimes associated with taking statins.
- **MIGRAINES.** Some research suggests that CoQ10 might decrease the frequency of these headaches.
- **PHYSICAL PERFORMANCE.** Because CoQ10 is involved in energy production, it's believed that this supplement might improve your physical performance. However, research in this area has produced mixed results.

Dosage is usually 30-200. Taking it twice a day seems to keep higher serum levels.

For just about anyone but certainly our patients with any cardiovascular issues:

RESVERATROL:

As a natural food ingredient, numerous studies have demonstrated that Resveratrol is a super antioxidant.

How Resveratrol helps:

- lowers blood pressure
- protects the brain
- lengthens life spans in animals
- decreases LDL and increases HDL
- increases insulin sensitivity
- eases joint pain
- Resveratrol also exhibits antitumor activity and is considered a potential candidate for the prevention and treatment of several types of cancer

Resveratrol has most often been used in doses of 250-1,000 mg by mouth daily for up to 3 months.

FOR JUST ABOUT ANYONE BUT CERTAINLY OUR PATIENTS WHO ARE EXERCISING REGULARLY OR THOSE WHO NEED HELP REPAIR THE GUT: AMINO ACIDS[1]

Amino acids, often referred to as the building blocks of proteins, are compounds that play many critical roles in your body. You need them for vital processes such as building proteins, hormones, and neurotransmitters. Amino acids are concentrated in protein-rich foods such as meat, fish, and soybeans.

Some people also take certain amino acids in supplement form as a natural way to boost athletic performance or improve mood. Amino acids are also critical in healing the lining of the gut.

Your body needs 20 different amino acids to grow and function properly. While all 20 of these are important for your health, only 9 are classified as essential, which, again, means that your body can't make them)

Here is a little more about the 9 essential amino acids, each of which perform several important jobs in your body:

1. **PHENYLALANINE.** Your body turns this amino acid into the neurotransmitters, tyrosine, dopamine, epinephrine, and norepinephrine. It plays an integral role in the structure and function of proteins and enzymes and the production of other amino acids.

2. **VALINE.** This is one of three branched-chain amino acids (BCAAs) on this list. That means it has a chain branching off from one side of its molecular structure. Valine helps stimulate muscle growth and regeneration and is involved in energy production.

---

1 https://www.healthline.com/nutrition/essential-amino-acids#how-many-are-there

3. **THREONINE.** This is a principal part of structural proteins, such as collagen and elastin, which are important components of your skin and connective tissue. It also plays a role in fat metabolism and immune function.

4. **TRYPTOPHAN.** Often associated with drowsiness, tryptophan is a precursor to serotonin, a neurotransmitter that regulates your appetite, sleep, and mood.

5. **METHIONINE.** This amino acid plays an important role in metabolism and detoxification. It's also necessary for tissue growth and the absorption of zinc and selenium, minerals that are vital to your health.

6. **LEUCINE.** Like valine, leucine is a BCAA that is critical for protein synthesis and muscle repair. It also helps regulate blood sugar levels, stimulates wound healing, and produces growth hormones.

7. **ISOLEUCINE.** The last of the three BCAAs, isoleucine is involved in muscle metabolism and is heavily concentrated in muscle tissue. It's also important for immune function, hemoglobin production, and energy regulation.

8. **LYSINE.** Lysine plays major roles in protein synthesis, calcium absorption, and the production of hormones and enzymes. It's also important for energy production, immune function, and the production of collagen and elastin.

9. **HISTIDINE.** Your body uses this amino acid to produce histamine, a neurotransmitter that is vital to immune response, digestion, sexual function, and sleep-wake cycles. It's critical for maintaining the myelin sheath, a protective barrier that surrounds your nerve cells.

Although your body can make nonessential amino acids, it cannot make essential amino acids, so you must get them from your diet. The best sources of essential amino acids are animal proteins such as meat, eggs, and poultry. However, some plant foods, such as the soy products, edamame, and tofu, contain all 9 essential amino acids. This means they are "complete" sources of protein. After you eat protein, your body breaks it down into amino acids and then uses them for various processes, such as building muscle and regulating immune function.

Our system needs amino acids for a variety of functions, including:

- creation and growth of connective tissue, and skin
- growth of muscle tissue and maintenance of muscle tone
- maintaining normal digestion
- providing energy for the body
- mood regulation by helping produce hormones
- helping with healthy skin, hair, and nails
- assisting athletes with endurance and pain tolerance during training and how the body perceives fatigue allowing them to perform longer before tiring out
- improving immune function
- helping develop lean muscle mass
- increasing overall strength
- helping with the production of antioxidants in the body to reduce cellular damage
- assisting with inflammation in the body
- helping the body metabolize fats especially when exercising

BCAAS: Of the 9 essential amino acids, 3 are the branched-chain amino acids (BCAAs): leucine, isoleucine, and valine. We can get BCAAs from protein-rich foods like eggs, meat, and dairy products. They are a popular dietary supplement especially with athletes and people who exercise a a lot. They are usually taken in powder form and are used to help with fatigue, improve athletic performance, and stimulate muscle recovery after exercise.

While amino acids are great for everyone, we especially recommend it to our patients who are regularly exercising. We recommend taking it either right before or right after a workout to help repair some of the damage done during exercises. Taking amino acid supplements may also be helpful for people who are healing after surgery.

FOR THE PATIENT THAT NEEDS MORE HELP IN THE REPLACE PHASE: DIGESTIVE ENZYMES

Digestive enzymes are proteins that help break down and digest. When digestion works as it should, it allows our body to absorb nutrients from food and give our body energy and fuel. Digestion starts at the mouth with saliva which starts breaking down food immediately. As the food moves through the body, there are points along the digestive process where enzymes are released and activated. These enzymes are made by your stomach, small intestine, and pancreas. You need these enzymes to break down carbohydrates, proteins, and fats. When our body doesn't make enough digestive enzymes, we can't break down certain foods, which means we can't get the needed nutrients from the food we eat. This is when we consider a supplement.Taking digestive enzymes as a supplement is not for everyone. Some people cannot tolerate these at first, so we do a few weeks of Remove before we start to Replace.

Please note that these must be taken with food. Here is a list of digestive enzymes we recommend to certain patients:

› pepsin
› bromelain
› lactase
› protease 1
› protease 2
› protease 3
› protease 4
› glucoamylase
› cellulase
› sucrase
› maltase
› phytase
› pectinase
› alpha-galactosidase
› lipase
› amylase 1

- amylase 2
- peptidase

FOR THE PATIENT THAT NEEDS HELP WITH GUT REPAIR AND JOINT REPAIR: COLLAGEN

Collagen is considered a complex protein because it is made up of 19 different amino acids. Collagen also makes up 90% of our connective tissue and bone mass and about 70% of our skin. However, as we reach our mid- to late twenties, our natural production slows down. When there is damage to the intestinal lining, these amino acids boost our body's natural ability to repair. Collagen protein has been found to help with healing stomach and intestinal lining. Collagen has also been found to help with joint healing in much the same way.

While this may seem like a lot, there are many more supplements available for a wide variety of issues. There are some we recommend using for cholesterol, diabetes, memory support, cardiovascular support, joint support, and mitochondrial support, but those are all very specific and are taken for very specific reasons. Once we get the diet straight and see what a patient is lacking for optimal health, only then do we create a supplement plan based on their very specific needs.

CHAPTER 7:

A QUICK RECAP

Okay, before we go any further, let's do a quick recap. This is the cliff notes summary of the entire book. Take a picture of it and give the book away.

You don't feel good.

The first thing you must do is go to your PCP and be fully checked out. Always rule out a disease first!

Once they tell you- "you're fine," you start using this book.

P.S. if they tell you that you're not fine, **LISTEN TO THEIR ADVICE** and use this book also so that your body can become stronger and more resilient so that you can manage the diagnosis.

Remember, just about everything you have going on that is making you feel horrible has to do with inflammation.

Your job is to get rid of the inflammation.

How do we do that? We start with the gut.

› Use the 4R Protocol: Remove, Replace, Reinnoculate, and Repair
› Use our REKNEW DIET
› Consider intermittent fasting
› Manage your stress, get some exercise, and get sleep.

If you feel better, you are done. Move on. Time to start a new Netflix series.

If you don't feel better after all of this, you may want to consider what we discuss in Chapters 8 and 9.

But don't start there, always start with the above.

Only go deep sea diving if the above fails.

CHAPTER 8:

MOVING INTO THE VORTEX: MOLD TESTING

Let me start by explaining that the following chapters on mold, hormones, and Lyme disease are just a very brief look into these topics. These chapters are not comprehensive coverage of these topics. In fact, each one of these topics needs its own book, let alone a chapter. But since I do have patients who have these issues, I felt that it was important that we at least give a brief overview so that you know where to go next if healing the gut didn't help you.

Most people who follow the protocol to fix their gut and adrenals will usually feel so much better and stop the search. This is great because it will save them time and money. Even if you are sure that mold is your issue, you STILL must follow the protocol to fix your gut because no provider should start treating you for mold unless you've already done that work. Treatment for mold is very hard on the body and should only be done if you are already working on your gut and your immune system so that you can handle the treatment. Cleaning your diet and repairing the gut is the foundation upon which we base the rest of the work.

That being said, let's talk about mold.

MOLD TOXICITY

Mold toxicity is more common than you might think. Most medical practitioners don't consider mold in their equation when a patient is unwell. As I said, this chapter is not even close to comprehensive, but if you really want to learn more, for a deep dive, the mold guru is Dr. Ritchie Shoemaker. He has a website called survivingmold.com. If you think you may have symptoms related to mold, this will be a great starting point for you.

Let me explain why mold is so bad. Well, it's only bad for some of us. Seventy-five percent of the population can be exposed to mold and never have an issue. Their body will excrete the mold and never have any symptoms, but for 25 percent of the population, there is a genetic makeup that makes it impossible for them to detox from mold exposure. The mold binds to their body and wreaks havoc.

Why?

So, now we have this foreign toxin in the body. For most of us, the immune system can fight this toxin off, but for some people, their bodies cannot make the antibodies necessary, and it accumulates.

Once in the system, the body sets up an inflammatory process. Without going into too much detail, this process then blocks certain normal pathways so that the body's immune system, neurological system, and endocrine system are affected. When the body is inflamed, it releases something called cytokines. One of the damaging effects of these cytokines is that they go to the hypothalamus, which controls the pituitary gland, the "master gland" that releases hormones.

The downstream effect of these cytokines on the pituitary gland is that it can affect just about every system in the body. This pathway affects adrenal hormones, sex hormones, thyroid hormones, kidney regulation, sleep disturbances, and leaky gut, which, as you know by now, will then trigger an autoimmune response. That's why people who are mold toxic can appear with all different kind of symptoms, which makes it hard to diagnose. This is also why treating the autoimmune issue, or the sex hormone issue, is not going to get the patient any better because those are the symptoms not the cause.

Here are some of the symptoms people suffering with mold toxicity may experience:

Pathognomonic Symptoms

(A pathognomonic symptom is one that is characteristic for the disease)

- › electric shock sensation
- › icepick-like pains
- › vibrating or pulsing sensation running up and down the spinal cord

Other possible symptoms

- › muscle weakness
- › numbness and tingling in different parts of the body
- › disequilibrium
- › dizziness
- › severe anxiety and depression
- › cognitive impairment
- › joint and muscle pain
- › headaches
- › GI symptoms
- › chest tightness and pain

How do we get it?

Mycotoxins (molds) can be inhaled, absorbed through our skin, or ingested in contaminated food. Dried fruit, aged cheeses, mushrooms, and processed meat can all produce mold in our system, but the major source is by being inhaled.

There are many types of molds including: Stachybotrys Aspergillus, Penicillium, Fusarium, Chaetomium, Alternaria, and Wallemia.

How do we test for mold?

Lab tests:

In general, when we test for inflammation in most patients, we use C reactive protein and sed rate (see Chapter 3) but for the mold patient, we need different markers. We would test to see if c4a TGF-beta-1 and MMP-9 and leptins are elevated and if VEGF, MSH and VIP are low.

The explanation of these tests is beyond the scope of this book but if you are interested to learn more, a great resource would be the book, *Toxic: Heal Your Body from Mold Toxicity, Lyme Disease, Multiple Chemical Sensitivities, and Chronic Environmental Illness* by Neil Nathan.

The good thing about these tests is that they can be run by conventional labs like Quest and Lab Corp and can be a good starting point. The downside is that these tests are not specific to mold. If they are abnormal, they can also indicate other infections such as Lyme or other parasites. So, to be sure that these abnormal symptoms are from mold, you will need specialized mold tests in specialty labs.

Real Time Laboratory and Great Plan Laboratory do urine testing for mold, which is very accurate. If you decide to do these tests, there is a recommendation to take glutathione 500mg twice a day for a week before the test. People with mold issues have these issues because their body is "holding onto" the mold. Taking the glutathione before the test helps "push" the mold into the urine and will give a more accurate result.

There are also screening tests that can be done at home called the Functional Acuity Test or FACT or the VCS test (Visual Contrast Sensitivity). You can go to the website, www.survivingmold.com, to get the VCS test done. This is a screening test, so a positive result is very suggestive of mold but if the results are negative and the symptoms persist, you should consider further testing.

What is the Treatment for Mold?

The treatment for mold toxicity is long and intense and again, beyond the scope of this book. But, to give you an idea of how it works, it involves taking something called "binders" which will bind to the mold and help the patient excrete the mold out. This process is hard on the body, especially for patients who are already unwell, which is why it is crucial that your diet, sleep, and exercise are on point as much as possible before embarking on this journey.

There are different protocols used by different medical providers, and the type of mold you have will be a factor as well. However, one thing is clear, you must remove yourself from the mold environment or remove the mold from your environment. Mold removal from an environment must be done by professionals, otherwise the cleaning process will release spores and make matters worse.

Dr. Ritchie Shoemaker, who is the pioneer of mold treatment, recommends using cholestyramine as the binder of choice. This is a medication that is used for cholesterol because it helps bind and remove cholesterol from the body. This medication binds to the toxins more strongly than the toxins bind to bile, so they can "pull" them out of the body and excrete them out. Details of this protocol are found in Dr. Shoemaker's book, *Mold Warriors: Fighting America's Hidden Health Threat.*

Dr. Joseph Brewer, another specialist in the treatment of mold, uses this binder as well but he also uses antifungal nasal sprays because he believes that the sinus and the gut are mostly colonized and need to be eradicated at the same time as binding. (You can find this information in Dr. Neil Nathan's book.)

There are different binders used for different toxins including:

- **OCHRATOXINS** – cholestyramine and activated charcoal

- **AFLATOXINS** – bound by activated charcoal and bentonite clay
- **TRICHOTHECENES** – bound by activated charcoal
- **GLIOTOXINS** – bound by bentonite clay and NAC (N-acetyl cysteine)

So, once again, if you are feeling unwell, you start with the recommendation in Chapter 7, and if you still have symptoms that fit the profile of someone with mold toxicity, you should very seriously consider testing. Mold can be very serious, and if left unresolved, can lead to greater health issues, and leave you in chronic pain and discomfort.

CHAPTER 9:

LYME DISEASE AND OTHER CO-INFECTION TESTING

WHAT ABOUT LYME DISEASE?

Let me start by saying that this is 100% NOT a comprehensive conversation about Lyme. Not. Even. Close. Lyme requires several books. However, I would be remiss if I didn't at least give you a cursory view of Lyme. Some of my patients who are persistently unwell are infected with Lyme and have chronic Lyme symptoms.

Lyme disease is a tick-borne disease. It's caused by a bacteria that is transferred from an animal to a human by a tick or a flea. These bacteria have been around for centuries, but why is that we see more people getting sick from this disease now more than ever?

Part of the answer is that our immune system's ability to keep this disease at bay has become compromised by the toxic environment in which we live. All Lyme-literate practitioners will tell you that you first must start with the gut when dealing with this problem. Lyme microbes thrive in unhealthy environments, so it is critical that we ensure that that the microbiome is balanced and that the liver is healthy enough to detoxify before we start treatment. So even if you have lyme, you gotta start with the gut.

There are two schools of thought regarding Lyme Disease. One is held by the Infectious Disease Society of America and one by the International Lyme and Associated Disease Society. The first school of thought believes that Lyme is as clear cut as any bacterial infection—you find it, you treat it—it's gone, end of story. The other school of thought presents that Lyme is anything but clear cut. They think that treating Lyme is very complex, and the disease is insidious and complicated. Personally, I agree with the second group.

Lyme disease is very complicated. Many doctors would like you to believe that it's as simple as diagnosing with a blood test and then treating it with antibiotics. You do a blood test, and if the results show that you are positive, you get treated with antibiotics and you are done. If your tests are negative, then you don't have Lyme.

Simple, right?

Nope. Lyme disease is about multiple, chronic infections that have long-term effects on the body's functions. It causes complex infections that then cause havoc on the immune system. It can affect the heart, the brain, and the nervous system. Lyme disease affects each person differently and intensely.

Initially, it was thought that Lyme disease was caused by one bacteria—borrelia burgdorferi—but we now know that there can be infections with borrelia, babesia, Bartonella and Ehrlichia organisms.

TESTING FOR LYME

If you suspect you have Lyme disease and regular lab testing is used, it's a bit of a gamble. If you are positive on a typical lab test, then you are positive. But if you are negative, Lyme cannot truly be ruled out. If you suspect Lyme disease due to possible exposure, and you are having symptoms that seem to fit the profile of the disease, do not stop investigating just because you received a negative Lyme test from your PCP. I strongly urge you to go to a

Lyme-literate medical provider and delve further into the problem.

Why is testing so difficult?

Simply put, the tests found in typical labs like LabCorp or Quest are just not comprehensive enough. There are several reasons for this.

1. The tests used by these labs are not designed to detect the exact bacteria you may have. For example, the tests are designed to detect a bacteria called Borrelia Burgdorferi and none of the other species that can also cause Lyme.

2. The typical labs tests approved by the FDA use a test called ELISA followed by another test called the Western Blot test. Both tests are designed to detect antibodies to Borellia Burgdorferi bacteria. Recent studies have shown that this type of testing can miss up to 60 percent of the bacteria present.

3. Additionally, these tests are called Indirect Tests, meaning they test the body's immune reaction to the bacteria but not actually the presence of the bacteria. However, the body may not have created antibodies to the bacteria if the test is done too early or if the patient's immune system hasn't created a response yet.

4. For those labs that do PCR testing, meaning they are looking for the bacterial DNA, they can also produce many negative results because the bacteria are sparse and may not be in the sample detected.

5. Some people have Lyme co-infections, meaning they don't have Lyme, so they test negative for Lyme disease. But they have the symptoms of Lyme, and it is due to the co-infection with a different type of bacteria that is not often tested for. They may have additional bacterial infections that do not cause Lyme. This is still an issue and needs to be addressed.

There are labs that can offer different options.

- **IGENEX** offers Lyme testing that includes many more species than just Borrelia Burgdorferi.
- **ADVANCE LABORATORY SERVICES** tests for borrelia culture test.

And there are other laboratories and other types of testing. The point is, don't let a negative lab result fool you. Continue to investigate if you are still experiencing symptoms that could lead to much bigger problems.

Symptoms

Some Lyme-literate doctors will diagnose based on symptoms. It's possible that people may be exposed to Lyme disease organisms for years but not become symptomatic until they experience a stressor later in life. Once that happens, the infections begin to gain an advantage over the immune system.

This explains why strengthening the immune system is key! There are certain symptom patterns that are associated with each kind of organism:

BABESIA OR BABESIA- LIKE ORGANISMS (BABLO)[2]

BABLO can affect the brain and nervous system. Patients will say they can't focus or think. Their mood is affected, and they are experiencing symptoms of depression and anxiety is common. Strong emotions and fear are dominant symptom of this.

Babesia can also affect the autonomic nervous system, which controls automatic functions of the body. So, it can cause POTS (postural orthostatic tachycardia syndrome) which causes a racing heartbeat like a pounding heart, especially at night. Babesia can also cause chills and sweats, insomnia, blurred vision, bowel motility issues, and bladder difficulty. Babesia does not usually cause pain, however.

2 Anderson, W. & Strasheim, C. 2016. New Paradigms in Lyme Disease Treatment. Lake Tahoe: BioMed Publishing Group

BARTONELLA OR BARTONELLA-LIKE ORGANISMS (BLO)

BLO can be transmitted by fleas on household pets. Usually, patients will come in and say, "You have to help me with my pain." They have pain in both the joints and the connective tissue around the joints and this pain will migrate to other areas of the body. They will also have recurring fevers, inflammation in the eyes, as well as skin issues.

BORRELIA

The most distinguishing feature of the symptoms people experience with Borrelia is that it causes fatigue. It can also cause pain, but the pain is more diffused.

You can see, however, that these symptoms are not specific and can be thought to be from other causes. This is especially true if you test negative for Lyme through a conventional lab. This explains why if you feel these symptoms are from lyme and you already did the work, went to your PCP, changed your diet, fixed your adrenals, etc., then it's time to test at different labs and consider going to a lyme-literate doctor.

TREATMENT

Treatment for Lyme Disease varies. For some people, if caught early enough, a course of antibiotics may do the trick. But unfortunately, most people are not diagnosed early on. For those people, antibiotics may not be enough. Additionally, for some patients who are already fragile, antibiotics may worsen their symptoms because of the havoc it causes to the microbiome.

There are some very well-known protocols for the treatment of Lyme. Here are just a few from these the lyme gurus:

› Dr. Dietrich Klinghart has a specific protocol which involves the use of certain herbs and natural antimicrobials. He tries to avoid antibiotics and prefers the use of Byron White Herbal Formulas.

- Dr. Neil Nathan feels that antibiotics are a necessary part of treatment, but he uses antibiotics in conjunction with herbal treatments and utilizes Stephen Buhner's herbal protocol.
- Dr. David Minkoff does not add antibiotics to his treatment protocol and espouses Intravenous Ozone and Silver treatments along with dietary recommendations and herbal antimicrobials.
- Dr. Raj Patel sometimes use antibiotics alone, sometimes herbal remedies alone, and other times, he will use a combination, all of which depends on the patient's needs and preferences.

The point is, the list of Lyme protocols is huge. Each one of these doctors have written their own body of work, and as I said earlier in this chapter, this is by no means an exhaustive piece on Lyme treatment. The goal is just to give you a starting point so that you can do your own research and find the protocol you like if indeed Lyme disease is the culprit. Despite their differences, one thing all these doctors and medical practitioners have in common is that they want their patients to be on healthy diets and take supplements that will strengthen their immune system. So, as you research these and other doctors and the many possible protocols, you can start the work with the cleaning up your diet.

CHAPTER 10:

HORMONE TESTING, FOOD TESTING, AND STOOL TESTING, OH MY!

These are three huge topics each deserving their own book series. I put them all here just so you can get a sense of what testing is available if you need to dig further

HORMONES

Many of my patients come in with symptoms they think are certain are related to their hormones. They are experiencing hot flashes, heart palpitations, night sweats and most of the time, it isn't their hormones. When these patients implement the diet changes, we recommend cleaning up their gut issues, the symptoms usually dissipate.

But there are times when hormones really are the issue at hand, especially for my older patients. Sometimes we need to dive a little deeper but remember, don't start here. Regardless, even if you're sure your issue is related to hormones, I still recommend that you start by addressing the diet. In my practice, we won't even consider hormone testing or treatment unless the patient is doing the work of repairing their gut issues first.

HORMONES: WHAT THEY DO AND HOW WE TEST

Hormones are chemicals secreted by glands and transported by the bloodstream throughout the body. Each hormone has its own purpose. When one of your hormone levels is not at the right level, too high or too low, it can throw the whole body out of whack.

If you are considering hormone testing, I recommend only testing through your saliva and only using Bioidentical Hormone Treatment (BHRT).

Let me explain why we uses these tests:

Saliva Testing

Your hormones circulate in the bloodstream by being bound to proteins that "carry" them along. When hormones are bound to protein, they get filtered through the salivary glands, so by testing the saliva, we can measure the hormones that are "bioavailable." Saliva testing lets us measure the amount of hormones that are free (unbound) and can act in the body. It lets us know if the levels are too high or too low. When levels are too high or low, this can create health issues like weight gain, irregular periods, and excess fatigue as well as other symptoms.

Testing saliva is the most non-invasive and stress-free way to test. All you do is spit into a sterile test tube, which then is sent to a lab. These samples are sent to the lab, the report is sent to your provider and the test results give a very clear picture of your hormone activity.

Saliva Testing should test the following hormones:

› **ESTRONE (E1)** – This is found in higher levels in post-menopausal women. The body makes this from body fat. Estrone is not used as a supplement.

› **ESTRADIOL (E2)** – This estrogen is the main one used during reproductive years. It is produced by ovaries. Estradiol levels decrease as women age and especially during menopause. It is used as a supplement to help with hot flashes, osteoporosis prevention, depression, anxiety, and reducing heart disease.

- **ESTRIOL (E3)** – This is a positive, mild-acting form of estrogen that is measured to aid control of hormone replacement therapy in menopausal women. It is especially helpful for the symptom of vaginal dryness and also has potential cancer prevention properties.
- **PROGESTERONE** – Progesterone plays an important role in fertility and pregnancy. For the post-menopausal woman, progesterone plays a great role in hot flashes and night sweats.
- **TESTOSTERONE** – This is an important hormone for men and for women. In men, it is produced by testes. In women, it is produced in the ovaries. It plays a role in bone health, body fat distribution, mood, sex drive, and many other functions.
- **DHEA** – DHEA (dehydroepiandrosterone) is a hormone produced by your body's adrenal glands. This is a hormone that breaks down into testosterone and estrogen. DHEA levels decline with age. Sometimes just supplementing with this is enough to get hormones levels in check.

Treatment

We recommend only using BHRT (Bioidentical Hormone Replacement Therapy). Bioidentical hormones are different from those used in traditional hormone replacement therapy (HRT) in that they're chemically identical to those our bodies produce naturally and are made from plant estrogens. The hormones used in traditional HRT are made from the urine of pregnant horses and other synthetic hormones.

Bioidentical hormones are available in the following forms:

- Patches
- Pills
- Gels
- Creams
- Injections

We prefer to use creams and pills in our in our practice. The common effects of reduced hormones are:

- Night sweats
- Vaginal dryness
- Hot flashes
- Pain during sex
- Fatigue
- Low sex drive
- Weight gain
- Problems sleeping
- Mood swings
- Memory loss
- Foggy thinking
- Loss of muscle mass

Remember, sometimes these symptoms resolve with lifestyle changes. So, don't assume that because you have these symptoms that it is hormones. If we determine that they are secondary to hormone issues, then you will notice an improvement in symptoms once you start replacing the hormones.

Additionally, for post-menopausal woman, not only is BHRT used to help with symptoms, studies have also shown that BHRT with estrogens is helpful in preventing or reducing osteoporosis and certain cancers. The point is, BHRT is not just for reducing symptoms, it also can help in the prevention of potential health issues. Most providers who are using BHRT are also using a compounding pharmacy that will custom make the hormone mixture that you need based on your individual hormone testing.

Since this is the only chapter that is recommending pharmaceuticals, I want to be sure that I tell you to educate yourself on this topic before embarking on it. Recommendations from national societies and medical experts state that people should consider the benefits and risks of both bioidentical and conventional hormones The United States Foods and Drug Administration (FDA) has endorsed some bioidentical hormones such as progesterone and bioidentical estriol, but the FDA has yet to approve compounded bioidentical hormones.

When you do your research, please note that the biggest opposition to small, custom-tailored compounding pharmacies are the big companies who produce hormones on a large scale. Draw your own conclusions here.

FOOD TESTING

There are times when we need to dig a little deeper into food testing. This is especially true If you have cleaned up your diet and feel that you are eating well but find that your symptoms aren't improving, especially with GI and skin issues.

Please be aware that these tests are expensive, so you only want to do these tests when they are really needed.

A Case Study: When Food Testing Helped

I had a patient whose gut and diet were super clean before she even came to me. We worked to clean up her diet even more. She was very thin and had no weight to lose. Despite all our efforts, her stomach was still a mess no matter what we did. She had GI symptoms even though her diet was super clean.

In this case, we decided to do food sensitivity testing for this patient. We discovered that spinach and tomatoes were irritating her system. These are two items we would have never considered removing from her diet were it not for her tests. Her symptoms improved greatly after removing these foods. Additionally, most people, who are at this level of sensitivity also need enzymes as described in Chapter 4, (Replace) so we started replacing her enzymes slowly, and she is now getting better.

Food sensitivity is NOT the same as food allergies.

There are true food allergies as well as sensitivities and intolerances. I will explain each one in detail below but here is a general overview.

FOOD ALLERGY: Immunologic hypersensitivity (IgE reaction) where your immune system responds quickly, like hives after eating a strawberry.

FOOD SENSITIVITY: Immunologic delayed reaction to food (IgG and IgA reactions) where your immune system responds much after exposure, like headaches a few days later after consuming nightshades.

FOOD INTOLERANCE: Non-Immunologic reaction to food where you have a response to the food, but it has nothing to do with an immune response. It's like gas and bloating after eating dairy.

The rest of this section about immunoglobulin is a level-one Nerd Alert. Feel free to totally skip it. It will not make a difference in your life.

> **NERD ALERT (Level-One):** Immunoglobulins (also known as antibodies) are proteins made by our immune system to fight antigens such as bacteria, viruses, and toxins. These antibodies are produced by our bodies in an immune system response to things we contact that the body recognizes as foreign (also called antigens), such as viral cells and bacteria. These antibodies are also able to respond to other foreign matter including pollen, dust, dander, and foods. Antibodies work to help the body fight against these "invaders."
>
> The body makes different immunoglobulins to combat different antigens. There are five classes of immunoglobulins, however, we are going to focus on the three that are relevant to us here.
>
> **IMMUNOGLOBULIN E (IGE)** - usually an immediate response to a foreign substance that has entered the body.
>
> **IMMUNOGLOBULIN G (IGG)** - usually food sensitivities that are less obvious and can last longer than an IgE allergy.
>
> **IMMUNOGLOBULIN A (IGA)** - plays a role in the immune function of mucous membranes.

IGE (IMMUNOGLOBULIN E) allergies

IgE (Immunoglobulin E) allergies are immediate responses to an antigen that has entered the body. This is your typical food allergy that many of us are familiar with. One example of an IgE response to a food allergy is with eggs. If a person with an egg allergy eats an omelette, the body thinks it's a foreign substance and creates an IgE response

After being exposed to this allergen, IgE antibodies to egg will stay in her body. When the person eats an egg again, the IgE antibodies will send out a reaction full of histamine and other compounds, which cause symptoms like inflammation and itching. This is where you see hives, itchiness, difficulty breathing, and other "typical" allergic reactions. This explains why antihistamines are used to calm this kind of reaction.

IgE food allergies usually do not go away but can decrease over time if an individual's health improves. The stronger the immune system and the healthier the gut, the better your body will be able to tolerate accidental exposure. In general, though, it's best to stay away from any food to which you are completely allergic.

IGE ALLERGY SYMPTOMS

Symptoms of an IgE allergy usually appear within seconds or minutes. These symptoms can include:

- Swelling/inflammation
- Hives/Rash
- Itching skin
- Difficulty breathing
- Throat tightening
- Anaphylactic shock (in severe cases)

IGE ALLERGY TESTING

IgE tests are done by most ENTs (ear, nose, throat) doctors or allergists. This can be done by a skin prick or patch testing.

IGG FOOD SENSITIVITIES

IgG (Immunoglobulin G) food allergies are delayed food allergies and are often called food "sensitivities." With IgG reactions, the immune system produces IgG antibodies, which can lead to inflammatory processes. Symptoms for IgG reactions can appear up to three days after the eating/drinking the problematic food.

Many people with IgG food sensitivities do not realize they have them for years, if not their entire lives. That's because the reaction shows up so many days later that it's hard to make the connection between the food and the reaction. Elimination of IgG-positive foods can often improve symptoms of irritable bowel syndrome, ADHD, and other autoimmune issues.

IGG ALLERGY SYMPTOMS

IgG antibodies create a different response. They don't release histamines, so you will not get the immediate hypersensitivity reactions of itching, hives, swelling, etc. This also means that antihistamines won't work here. Symptoms of an IgG reaction can appear up to 72 hours after eating a food. These symptoms can include:

- Anxiety
- Headaches
- Nausea
- Depression
- Bloating/gas
- Diarrhea
- Constipation
- Acid reflux
- Joint aches
- Fatigue
- Mood changes
- Hyperactivity
- Loss of breath
- Weakness

- Brain fog/memory issues

Certain conditions can arise from food sensitivities such as:

- Arthritis
- Migraines
- Ear Infections
- Eczema
- Sinusitis
- Asthma
- Colitis

What this means is that the headache and migraines that you have had all your life or the eczema that won't go away may be a food sensitivity. And even though you have gone to an allergist, and they found nothing, remember that they typically only do IgE testing.

IGG AND LEAKY GUT

IgG sensitivities are often associated with many digestive problems including leaky gut (aka intestinal permeability). (See Chapter 3 for more on leaky gut.)

Leaky gut may trigger inflammation and changes in our good gut bacteria. Chronic, prolonged inflammation and toxicity can be a cause of autoimmune disease and other related disorders.

IGG TESTING AND ELIMINATION DIET

It is often difficult to pinpoint exactly which food(s) cause problems because of the delayed appearance of IgG symptoms. Because of this, we recommend an elimination diet. This is the cheapest way to get to your answers—eliminate the foods, watch the symptoms improve and then methodically reintroduce. But there are tests that can be done to make this process much shorter, and these are IgG tests. However, conventional labs do not do these tests. The labs that do this testing are Genova, Great Plain or Cyrex. We tend to use Cyrex in our practice.

Once you know the foods that your body will have a reaction to, an elimination diet follows to avoid foods for a certain time (usually about three months). Take this time to heal (replace, reinnoculate and repair). Food sensitivities can improve, and you may be able to reintroduce some of the foods back into your life.

IGA REACTIONS

While IgA reactions are not directly related to food allergies and sensitivities, we talked about leaky gut just briefly here, so I thought I'd mention another test having to do with intestinal permeability.

IgA (Immunoglobulin A)/Secretory IgA (sIgA) is found in high concentrations in the mucous membranes like those which line the respiratory passages and gastrointestinal tract. Secretory IgA (sIgA) provides protection against potentially harmful microbes. It is the body's first line of defense against bacteria, food particles, parasites, and viruses. Chronic stress, frequent antibiotic use, as well as an overload of foods like soda, coffee, alcohol, or sugar can thin the lining of the gut.

SIGA TESTING

A Secretory IgA (SIgA) test checks to see how strong your gut lining is. This will show a person's ability to defend against infections, allergies, and food reactions as well as provide insight into next steps in the treatment of health issues. These tests can be done in a regular lab. It will not be food-specific, but it will give an overall sense of how "angry" your belly is.

FOOD INTOLERANCES

While food allergies trigger the immune system, food intolerances do not. A food intolerance, however, can cause some of the same symptoms as a food allergy/sensitivity, so people often get them confused.

Food intolerances are usually caused by a deficiency/absence of an enzyme needed to digest/process a food. For example:

People with lactose intolerance do not have enough of the enzyme lactase that is needed to break down the sugar lactose found in cow's milk.

People with a histamine intolerance could be lacking the DAO or HNMT enzymes, which lead to an excess of histamine.

Histamine is a chemical found in some of the body's cells that can cause many of the symptoms of allergies, like a runny nose or sneezing. Histamine intolerance is a little different than other food intolerances because of the buildup of histamine. It's best to stay away from certain foods until histamine is lowered.

Some foods to avoid if you have a histamine intolerance may include:

- alcohol
- fermented beverages
- fermented foods
- dairy products including yogurt
- sauerkraut
- dried fruits
- avocados
- eggplant
- spinach
- processed or smoked meats
- shellfish
- aged cheese

FOOD INTOLERANCE TESTING

Food intolerances do not have a specific blood test because the immune system is not involved, and immunoglobulins will not be present in the blood. It's one of those things you can only figure out through trial and error.

STOOL TESTING

Again, we only use this "fun" test when we are running out of ideas to help certain patients significantly improve their health or reduce their symptoms. And we venture into this territory only after the patient has followed our protocols and still has not improved.

As I have said many times, always start with the basics. Change the diet and see how far you get. If you still have GI symptoms, stool testing is a possible way to go. When we do food testing, we want to see what the body is reacting to and consider removing those items from our diet. But what if our GI has some sort of infection or imbalance in good/bad bacteria (dysbiosis)? That's when stool testing is effective. We like to use a test called the GI Effects Comprehensive Stool Profile from a company called Genova. Here is how they describe the test on their website:

Nerd Alert: GI EFFECTS COMPREHENSIVE STOOL PROFILE
(https://www.gdx.net/)

The GI Effects Comprehensive Stool Profile can reveal important information about the root cause of many common gastrointestinal symptoms such as gas, bloating, indigestion, abdominal pain, diarrhea, and constipation. This stool analysis utilizes biomarkers such as fecal calprotectin to differentiate between Inflammatory Bowel Disease (IBD) and Irritable Bowel Syndrome (IBS) In addition, Genova's GI Effects test can be used to evaluate patients with a clinical history that suggests a gastrointestinal infection or dysbiosis.

Gut microbes are codependent with one another and with their human host, and the health of one affects the other. A sizeable volume of research associates a dysbiotic, or imbalanced gut microbiome, with multiple disease states both within and outside of the GI tract. The diverse metabolic activities of the microbiome ultimately impact the human host, and the activities of the human host ultimately affect the health of their microbiome.

The GI Effects Comprehensive Stool Profile Biomarkers

The biomarkers on the GI Effects Comprehensive Profile reflect the three key functions of gut health arranged in the "DIG" format: Digestion/Absorption, Inflammation/Immunology, and the Gut Microbiome:

Digestion/Absorption:

PANCREATIC ELASTASE-1 is a marker of exocrine pancreatic function.

PRODUCTS OF PROTEIN BREAKDOWN are markers of undigested protein reaching the colon.

FECAL FAT is a marker of fat breakdown and absorption.

Inflammation/Immunology:

CALPROTECTIN is a marker of neutrophil-driven inflammation. Produced in abundance at sites of inflammation, this biomarker has been proven clinically useful in differentiating between Inflammatory Bowel Disease (IBD) and Irritable Bowel Syndrome (IBS).

EOSINOPHIL PROTEIN X is a marker of eosinophil-driven inflammation and allergic response.

FECAL SECRETORY IGA is a marker of gut secretory immunity and barrier function.

FECAL OCCULT BLOOD TEST detects hidden blood. Fecal immunochemical testing (FIT) has been recommended by the American College of Gastroenterology as the preferred noninvasive test for colorectal cancer screening/detection.

Gut Microbiome:

METABOLIC INDICATORS include short-chain fatty acids and beta-glucuronidase, demonstrate specific and vital metabolic functions performed by the microbiota.

COMMENSAL BACTERIA demonstrate the composition and relative abundance of gut organisms.

More than 95% of commensal gut organisms are anaerobic and are difficult to recover by traditional (aerobic) culture techniques.

GI Effects assesses a set of 24 genera/species that map to 7 major phyla.

BACTERIAL AND MYCOLOGY CULTURES demonstrate the presence of specific beneficial and pathological organisms.

BACTERIAL AND MYCOLOGY SENSITIVITIES are provided for pathogenic or potentially pathogenic organisms that have been cultured. The report includes effective prescriptive and natural agents.

PARASITOLOGY includes comprehensive testing for all parasites on every parasitology exam ordered.

GI Effects provides microscopic fecal specimen examination for ova and parasites (O&P), the gold standard of diagnosis for many parasites.

6 Polymerase Chain Reaction (PCR) targets detect common protozoan parasites including Blastocystis spp, Cryptosporidium parvum/hominis, Cyclospora cayetanensis, Dientamoeba fragilis, Entamoeba histolytica, and Giardia. PCR for organisms is emerging as a highly sensitive method for infectious organism detection.

Selection of a one-day or three-day sample collection is based on the clinician's clinical index of suspicion for parasitic infection. If there is no/low suspicion, a one-day sample will likely be adequate. For high suspicion, a three-day sample collection is optimal.

Additional Biomarkers Available:

- Campylobacter
- Clostridium difficile
- Escherichia coli
- Fecal Lactoferrin
- Helicobacter pylori
- Macro Exam for Worms
- Zonulin Family Peptide
- KOH Preparation for Yeast

The bottom line is that this stool test gives us A LOT of information about what's happening in your gut—from the source! We use Genova Labs, and they send us a very detailed report on what is going on with the patient's gut, and they also offer suggestions on how to treat it, which we take into consideration as we put our patient plan together. Again, these tests are expensive, and we recommend only using them once you've tried the "free" stuff first.

CHAPTER 11:

THE KNEW METHOD:

OUR APPROACH TO BETTER HEALTH

I hope by this point my message is clear—you can do this on your own. You can be the Game Changer in your own life. Follow the 4R protocol, check out my recommendations in the Appendix and get yourself feeling better. That said, it is always great to have a guide to work with you and customize a plan that is just right for you specifically.

For those of you who are interested in working with me and my team, I decided to write this chapter to give you an overview of my signature process—The Knew Method—and tell you what it's all about. The Knew Method is designed to empower patients to realize that their symptoms are not in their head because you always KNEW there was a better way.

If you read Chapter 1, (even though I said you didn't have to) you know the story of my wife and I and how we came to the world of functional medicine. If you didn't read that chapter, you might want to go back and check it out. It's a good story, and it leads to why I believe so wholeheartedly in what we offer here at The Knew Method.

What Gina and I discovered through her health journey, in addition to what I learned through my education and in working with my patients, led me to create this program. This approach drastically changed our lives and allowed me to help so many others from a range of people who are not feeling optimal to those who are suffering greatly with various diseases.

I'm a methodical person. I like to be organized and have data at my fingertips. So, I took everything I learned and created a system that I can use for my patients to ensure that I address every patient's needs and tailor it to their specific issues.

HOW DOES IT WORK?

We start with a consultation with someone on my team. It's a quick "get to know each other" so we can see if we are a good fit for each other. If everything goes well, we schedule you for our Discovery Session. This is a one-hour session with me.

Prior to this meeting, there is some homework we both must do. You will be given a very detailed questionnaire. This is your opportunity to tell your whole story. My team will order specific blood tests and of course, we will order a saliva test for adrenal fatigue. Once we have your answers, the blood and saliva results, I will prepare for our meeting where we will discuss the results.

During our meeting, we will go over everything in detail and discover what is happening and making you feel unwell. My goal in this meeting is to show you that "it's not in your head." I will show you what I see from my unique perspective so that you can finally understand what's going on.

After our session, you will be equipped with understanding the "why" behind what you are feeling and get a general sense of what you need to do next. This may be enough for you, and you may refer back to this book and start doing the work on your own. If, however, you want us to help you on the journey and create a customized plan for you, then you can opt to work with me and my team. We insist that our patients commit to a year-long program. I don't believe that anything long lasting happens in a 30-60-90-day program. Real change takes time. Moreover, as we work together, we will discover new issues that come up; one of my recent patients called it peeling an onion.

THE KNEW METHOD PROGRAM:

As I mentioned, The Knew Method is a year-long program and is designed to help you create your own change and optimize your health. This method is designed to balance your gut health, remove toxins, and start reversing your symptoms. The goal is to reset your health and get you on track to feeling better, having more energy, and enjoying what you love with the people you love.

Here is what the 12-month program consists of:

- **A complete customized nutrition guide**

  This is created for and with you and is customized directly to your individual needs and health issues.

- **Monthly Consultations with Dr. E (that's me) for the entire year**

  Every month, we will track your symptoms using our state-of-the-art software. You will meet with Dr. E once a month to evaluate your progress and adjust things accordingly. Together, you will create a new plan for each month.

- **5 IV Vitamin Infusions**

  Our signature infusions are gamechangers for your health. For those of you who live far away or are needle phobic, we can replace this part with oral supplements.

- **Weekly Virtual Check-Ins with a Health Coach**

  You will be connected to your own health coach for weekly check-ins for the entire year. We know that the critical piece in making these lifestyle changes is consistent support. These calls help with questions that come up and address any challenges that arise so that you can stay on course with your customized plan.

- **Lifestyle Guidance on stress, sleep, exercise**

  We have tools to help you reduce stress, sleep better, and get the right exercise plan in place.

- **Supplements** *that were handpicked for you based on your needs. These may change monthly depending on where you are on your journey.*

- **Access to our members only #GameChanger Facebook Group**

  Support from fellow gamechangers is ... well, a game changer. It's good to know that there are lots of people working with us that can cheer you on and help you stay on the path to feeling better. It's a community of people who all want to see each other living healthier and happier lives. Videos and Facebook Lives from Dr. E will also provide support and important information.

- **VIP email access for same day issues/concerns**

  We're here for you. If you need to reach out to ask a question or to get some immediate support, you will be able to reach us and get a response in less than 24 hours.

- **Updating nutrition goals monthly**

  Tracking progress, seeing what is working for you or what needs to be changed or tweaked to make sure your nutritional goals are met is all part of the service at The Knew Method.

- **25% off all IVs and supplements**

  Because you are a member of The Knew Method community, we offer you substantial discounts on all IVs and supplements as needed.

- **Monthly symptom tracking**

  This is a huge part of The Knew Method. Our unique software allows us to track improvements or changes in your symptoms, so we know what to tweak, change, or remove from your diet or the supplements you're on by tracking your symptoms each month.

- **Bi-monthly bloodwork**

  Every other month, we will repeat bloodwork and assess changes, so we continue to improve your health.

Remember, you can do much of this on your own, we also offer membership with instructional videos for those of you who want to try this on your own with TheKnewMethod.com/courses.

For those of you who are all in and ready to take it to the next level and want that one-on-one service, you can book a consult with us here TheKnewMethod.com/consult. Working with me and my team is not for everyone. It's only for those of you who are ready to do the work and make the change. If you are ready to #CreateYou-rOwnChange and do what it takes to be a #GameChanger, then we would love to work with you.

FINAL WORD

Through my work as an NP, I have the privilege of taking care of thousands of patients. Through the businesses I create, I have the honor of helping and empowering the people who work with me. My mission is to help and empower people whenever I can. This book as an extension of this mission.

It is my deepest hope that this book helps you find a path to gain control of your health destiny and become the game changer in your life.

APPENDIX 1

REKNEW FOOD PLAN

If you are ready to change how you feel, get started today!

We suggest the ReKnew Diet to help our patients feel better *faster*. It may feel restrictive at first, but it is designed to give you results in a short amount of time so that you can begin to heal your gut. After the initial difficulty, your body will likely get used to the diet and your cravings will lessen.

Remember, it is meant to be used as a first step not as a "forever" diet (so don't panic). This plan removes the foods that commonly cause inflammation and focuses on adding foods that are restorative and detoxifying. It aims to regulate your blood sugar and balance your hormones. Patients following The ReKnew Food Plan usually experience improved cognition/mood, less pain, less fatigue, more energy, better quality of sleep, and generally even weight loss. The latest scientific research suggests that there is a correlation be tween the foods we now eat (Standard American Diet) and the tendency toward inflammation in the body and autoimmune and chronic illnesses. The chemicals that are added to foods, particularly in processed foods, will cause inflammation in the gut. When the intestines become inflamed, our ability to absorb nutrients is compromised. If we eliminate certain foods and replace them with natural, whole foods, in time we can reduce the inflammation in the body.

HOW CAN I START THE REKNEW FOOD PLAN?

Start the ReKnew Food Plan by removing these four food groups from your diet: Sugar, Grains, Legumes, and Dairy. Foods that contain gluten, grains, sweeteners, and dairy products must be removed for the gut to heal and allow the immune system to begin to work properly again. While you remove those food groups it is critical that you also add whole foods to your diet. Whole foods will help with detoxification and provide nutritional support that you need to heal from inside out. We recommend this diet in combination with our method for Intermittent Fasting, the 16:8 method. The ReKnew Food Plan is not about feeling deprived. It is about healing the gut and getting you feeling great!

FEATURES OF THE REKNEW FOOD PLAN:

Removing Sugar:

Sugar is everywhere. Not only is it found in sweet foods, it's found in ketchups, nutritional bars, and so many other hidden places. It is deliberately put into these foods because the brain will crave more and we will consume more. However, when we eat a diet that contains too much sugar, we run the risk of developing autoimmune, gastrointestinal, neurological and other chronic health issues. The ReKnew Food Plan is designed to help reset the system to lower inflammation and prevent and improve chronic issues.

Removing Processed Foods:

If you want to know if a food is processed, look at the ingredient list—if there are ingredients that would never make it into a household kitchen—its processed. Don't be fooled. No matter how many vitamins and nutrients these products are said to contain, they offer no nutritional value. Companies purposely "fortify" foods with vitamins to confuse the consumer. A healthy diet needs to consists of clean, fresh, whole foods.

When it comes to processed foods, two good rules of thumb are:

› Don't eat anything that is incapable of rotting.
› If it comes from a plant, eat it; if it was made in a plant, don't.

Removing Dairy and Grain:

Gluten sensitivity causes changes in the gut that leads to inflammation, which can lead to chronic health issues. This is true for many people even if they don't have celiac disease. Dairy isn't the superfood that it's claimed to be. It causes inflammation even in people who are not lactose intolerant. Part of the issue is in how we process our gluten and dairy in a modern society. Removing these two food groups should make a significant change in how you feel and will impact your health greatly.

When following the ReKnew Food Plan, keep it simple. Think of it this way, if you can make it in your kitchen (or someone else's kitchen for those of you who don't like to cook), it's safe to eat. But if you need a degree in chemistry to understand the ingredients don't put it in your body. Adding low glycemic fruits, non starchy vegetables, meat, poultry, and fish will give you the nutrients you need to heal from the inside out. Eat the rainbow by trying vegetables of different colors.

APPENDIX 2

INTERMITTENT FASTING

Before we get into the nitty gritty of how to do Intermittent Fasting, I want to give you a little bit of a background as to why Intermittent Fasting is so good for you.

By design, we can go for hours without eating. Fasting is a practice that has been around throughout time because there were no refrigerators and there was no DoorDash or UberEats. That means sometimes there was food, and sometimes there wasn't. As long as you weren't dehydrated and had access to water, you were good. You could go for hours, if not days, without eating. And guess what, the species survived and thrived.

How is it possible that we can go for hours without eating? Let's dig into why that is. Every process in our body needs glucose, and everything that we eat gets broken down into glucose. There are two ways we can get glucose. 1) We eat something our body converts into glucose and 2) The body can convert fat into glucose (a process called gluconeogenesis).

You already know how to do the first one (just eat). The second way of getting glucose only happens when we fast. So, if you reach for food every few hours, you will never turn this cool feature on.

"Okay, that's cool, but why do I feel so shaky in between meals?" That's because your body has never used this feature and doesn't know how to go without food for extended amounts of time. You constantly need refueling. If you had a car that needed a refill every few hours, well, you would want to switch it to a more fuel-efficient car, right? Once you learn how to fast, your body will be able to switch between periods of getting food and without that shaky feeling. But, like everything, it takes practice.

"Okay, but why should I bother, what's so great about it?" Bottom line—it reduces inflammation. It's basically spring cleaning for your body. During a fast, you get a clean-up crew that repairs, removes and reduces inflammation.

INTERMITTENT FASTING CAN ALSO:

- Help reduce the risk of heart disease
- Lower the risk of diabetes
- Improve sleep quality
- Increase insulin sensitivity
- Help reduce bad cholesterol (LDL)
- Break down triglycerides
- Induce various cellular repair processes
- Help prevent Alzheimer's disease
- Help with weight loss
- Increase brain function

Of course, this is just one tool in an overall healthy lifestyle that will help us get to our goals. I want to be clear that I am not saying that Intermittent Fasting is going to cure your cancer or reverse Alzheimer's. There are no quick fixes! I'm just saying that this is one tool that you have in your toolbox, to help with prevention and improvement.

HOW TO GET STARTED WITH INTERMITTENT FASTING

CHOOSE A 16:8 TIMEFRAME THAT WORKS FOR YOU. Choose a timeframe that best fits into your schedule. The very first thing you must do is pick a timeframe that works for you, not one that works for them or for her or for him.

DO NOT TRY TO FORCE INTERMITTENT FASTING OVERNIGHT. Listen to your body. If you are shaky or hangry, eat. For those of you just starting out, it is hard to get to those 16 hours at first. Don't push yourself. The last thing you want to be is shaky and hangry and feeling like you're going to pass out. This is a marathon, not a sprint. Get there slowly.

FOR THOSE OF YOU WHO ALREADY EXCEL AT 16 HOURS, TRY 18 HOURS.

DON'T FORGET TO HYDRATE. Remember to drink water, flavored seltzer, black tea or black coffee—they do not break your fast. These liquids are your friends.

WHEN IT IS FINALLY TIME TO EAT, MAKE GOOD, SOLID CHOICES. You don't want to ruin everything you just did by hitting a big box of donuts or a whole pizza pie. Choose good whole foods that make sense to eat while you are on this health mission. Ideally, choose foods from the Reknew Diet.

APPENDIX 3

THE FOUR R'S:

REMOVE

Remove the factors that negatively impact your GI tract and your whole system. Remove inflammatory foods and pathogens.

REPLACE

Add good nutrient filled food (eat the rainbow) and digestive enzymes if needed.

REINNOCULATE

Reintroducing good bacteria or probiotics into your gut to create a more balanced gut flora and microbiome.

REPAIR

Repair the lining of your gut with supportive food and nutrients.

APPENDIX 4

RECOMMENDED LAB TESTS

GENERAL BLOOD WORK

CBC (Complete Blood Count)

WHAT: This is a test to let us know how your blood cells and platelets are doing.

WHY: CBC gives us information on anemia, clotting and certain blood cancers.

CMP (Comprehensive Metabolic Panel)

WHAT: The CMP test measures 14 different substances in your blood which allows us to evaluate kidney function, liver function and blood sugar and electrolyte levels.

WHY: Used to inform us about the body's chemical balance, energy use, and metabolism.

HEMOGLOBIN A1C

WHAT: This tests the average level of blood sugar in a patient for the three months prior to taking the test.

WHY: Often used to diagnose prediabetes and diabetes.

VITAMIN D

WHAT: A test to measure how much vitamin D is in the body.

WHY: Vitamin D is needed for, immune function, and protecting bone, muscle, and heart health and so much more.

STANDARD LIPID PANEL

WHAT: This blood test is commonly used to monitor and screen for risk of cardiovascular disease and includes three measurements of cholesterol levels and a measurement of the triglycerides.

WHY: Important for assessing the cardiovascular health of a patient.

VITAMIN B12 AND FOLATE

WHAT: A test to check B12 and Folate levels.

WHY: Vitamin B12 is a nutrient that helps keep your nerve cells healthy and helps make DNA. It is a key part of your energy and mood.

IRON PANEL WITH TIBC AND FERRITIN

WHAT: These tests measure the levels of iron in the system

WHY: Iron and ferritin levels are important for managing anemia and other blood issues. Ferritin can also be used as a sign of inflammation

VItamin A (Retinol)

WHAT: This test is to evaluate the level of Vitamin A in the system.

WHY: Vitamin A is important for normal vision, the immune system, and reproduction. Vitamin A also helps the heart, lungs, kidneys, and other organs work properly.

TSH

WHAT: This test measures the thyroid-stimulating hormone.

WHY: Higher levels might mean an underactive thyroid. Lower levels an overactive thyroid.

T3 Uptake, T4 (Thyroxine) Total, Free T4 Index (T7), T3 Free

WHAT: This test is used to assess the hormones produced by the thyroid.

WHY: The test gives us more detailed information on how the thyroid is working. For example, the thyroid might be making enough T4, but it may not be converting to T3 which will require a different.

Urinalysis

WHAT: Tests the urine sample to screen for urinary tract infections, kidney issues, and diabetes.

WHY: This should be part of a routine checkup or because it may be a red flag for some silent issues happening in the body.

MORE COMPREHENSIVE STUDIES

Liver Info

Hepatic Function Panel

(Total Protein, Albumin, Globulin (calc), Albumin/Globulin Ratio (calc), Total Bilirubin, Direct Bilirubin, Indirect Bilirubin (calc), Alkaline Phosphatase, AST, ALT), GGT

WHAT: This a blood test that checks for liver injury, infection, or disease.

WHY: The liver processes just about everything we take and it's critical that we know how it is functioning.

More Thyroid

Thyroid Peroxidase (TPO)

WHAT: This test detects TPO antibodies in the blood.

WHY: We do this test when a patient has been diagnosed with thyroid disease to help determine if patients have an autoimmune issue.

Thyroglobulin Antibodies

WHAT: This test measures the amount of Immunoglobin antibodies in the blood.

WHY: We do this test because high levels can be an indicator of the autoimmune disorder in the thyroid.

TRAB (thryotropin receptor antibodies)

WHAT: This blood test helps diagnose the autoimmune thyroid condition known as Graves' Disease.

WHY: To determine if the patient is dealing with this disease and begin a treatment plan.

TSI (Thyroid stimulating immunoglobulin)

WHAT: This test measures the amount of Immunoglobin in the blood to see signs of an overactive thyroid. TSIs which are the antibodies that inform the thyroid gland that it needs to become more active.

WHY: We do this test because high levels can be an indicator of the autoimmune disorder Graves' disease, which can lead to other autoimmune issues in the future.

OTHER

Magnesium

WHAT: This test measures the amount of magnesium in the blood.

WHY: Magnesium plays many crucial roles in the body, such as supporting muscle and nerve function and energy production. Low mag levels can often cause muscle spasms and constipation.

C-Peptide

WHAT: The C-peptide test lets us determine if the body is producing insulin.

WHY: A high level of C-peptide can mean your body is making too much insulin. It may be a sign of type 2 diabetes and/or Insulin resistance.

HS CRP

WHAT: This test is used as a marker for inflammation.

WHY: This level goes up in response to an infection, autoimmune disease or other systemic damage that may be occurring.

CELIAC TESTING

Celiac Disease Comprehensive Panel

Tissue Transglutaminase Antibody

WHAT: Tissue transglutaminase is an enzyme that fixes damage in your body.

People with celiac disease often make antibodies that attack this enzyme. These are called anti-tissue transglutaminase antibodies.

WHY: It is one of several blood tests that may be used to help diagnose celiac disease.

IgA (Immunoglobulin A)

WHAT: immunoglobulin A (IgA) is an antibody that's part of your immune system. IgA is found in mucous membranes, especially in the respiratory and digestive tracts.

WHY: High levels of IGA can A Signal of Chronic Inflammation/ Infection.

HLA Typing for Celiac Disease

WHAT: Celiac disease is strongly associated with the HLA gene. Approximately 90% of celiac patients express the HLA-DQ2.

WHY: Genetic Test to see if there is a likelihood of celiac disease This test does not diagnose celiac disease but if positive can suggest the person is genetically likely to have it.

HORMONES

FSH and LH

WHAT: Luteinizing hormone (LH) and follicle-stimulating hormone (FSH) are called gonadotropins because stimulate the gonads - in males, the testes, and in females, the ovaries.

WHY: The levels vary depending on the age. It helps determine reproductive issues and also used to determine menopause.

Prolactin

WHAT: The prolactin test measures this hormone in the blood which is released by the pituitary gland.

WHY: In women, too much prolactin can also cause menstrual problems and infertility (the inability to get pregnant). In men, it can lead to lower sex drive and erectile dysfunction (ED).

Testosterone Free and Total

WHAT: This test measures the level of bioavailable testosterone and total testosterone levels.

WHY: Testosterone levels are connected to fatigue, weight gain, decreased drive and many other symptoms for both men and women.

AUTOIMMUNE

Lyme Disease AB w/Reflex (IGG, IGM)

WHAT: A test to determine if there are antibodies in the patient's system that are indicators of the presence of Lyme Disease.

WHY: We do this test to assess if the person has Lyme disease and determine next steps.

ANA Screen, Antinuclear Antibody Test

WHAT: This test looks for certain antibodies in your body.

WHY: A positive result can mean the presence of autoimmune diseases A positive test for antinuclear antibodies (ANA) does not, by itself, indicate the presence of an autoimmune disease.

SED Rate

WHAT: A way to measure the inflammation.

WHY: A high sed rate is a general nonspecific test that indicates if there is inflammation in the body.

Uric Acid

WHAT: A way to measure amount of uric acid in the urine or blood.

WHY: We do this test to check for high uric acid levels. If too much uric acid stays in the body, it can cause crystals to form which can settle in the joints and cause gout, a form of arthritis that can be very painful.

Rheumatoid Factor

WHAT: This test measures the amount of rheumatoid factor (proteins produced by your immune system) in the blood.

WHY: High RF levels in the blood can indicate an autoimmune condition, such as rheumatoid arthritis.

Sjögren's Antibody (SS-A, SS-B)

WHAT: A way to test the blood for very specific antibodies related to Sjögren's.

WHY: Sjögren's Antibody (SS-B) is present only if Sjögren's Antibody (SS-A) is also detected. The presence of both antibodies (SS-A and SS-B) strengthen the diagnosis of Sjögren's Syndrome.

DNA (DS) Antibody

WHAT: This is a DNA blood test we use to help formulate the diagnosis of lupus as a possibility.

WHY: A high level of anti-dsDNA in the blood is strongly associated with lupus and is often significantly increased during or just prior to a flare-up.

SM Antibody - SM/RNP Antibody

WHAT: This test looks for smooth muscle antibodies (SMAs) in the blood. A smooth muscle antibody (SMA) is a type of antibody known as an autoantibody.

WHY: Sm antibodies are a specific serum marker for systemic lupus erythematosus (SLE), and high levels can be linked to mixed connective tissue disorder.

Cyclic Citrullinated Peptide AB (CCP IGG)

WHAT: A test to detect and measure CCP antibodies in the blood which are produced by the immune system and sometimes attack healthy tissues by mistake.

WHY: We do this test to help diagnose rheumatoid arthritis. If the test comes back positive, it may indicate rheumatoid arthritis.

C-Reactive Protein

WHAT: This test is to assess health conditions likely associated with inflammation including autoimmune diseases.

WHY: A high level of CRP in the blood is a marker for inflammation.

GENETIC TESTING

Methylenetetrahydrofolate Reductase (MTHFR)

WHAT: This test is used to find out if the patient has one of two MTHFR mutations: C677T and A1298C Which affects methylation. Methylation is is how your body transfers one set of atoms into a series of amino acids, proteins, enzymes, and DNA in each cell and tissue in your body.

WHY: Methyl groups in your body are the 'on-off' switches of the cells' activities. Which are responsible for all tissues and organs in the body, it is vital they are healthy and working as optimally as possible.

APOE Genotype

WHAT: This test is to detect the presence of the APOE4 variant, which is associated with increased risk of late-onset (age >60-65) Alzheimer's disease.

WHY: Having the gene does guarantee that someone will develop Alzheimer's, steps can be taken to reduce the risk.

INSULIN RESISTANCE SCORE

Cardio IQ(R) Insulin Resistance Panel with Score

WHAT: This is a special test panel run by Quest we do to see if a patient is insulin resistant.

WHY: Insulin resistance is a cause of inflammation. This panel can detect insulin resistance much earlier than a typical A1C test can.

APPENDIX 5

BOOKS I RECOMMEND

The Disease Delusion: *Conquering the Causes of Chronic Illness for a Healthier, Longer, and Happier Life*
Dr. Jeffrey S. Bland

Healing Lyme: *Natural Healing of Lyme Borreliosis and the Coinfections Chlamydia and Spotted Fever Rickettsiosis*
Stephen Harrod Buhner

The Inflammation Syndrome: *Your Nutrition Plan for Great Health, Weight Loss, and Pain-Free Living*
Jack Challem

Find Your Food Triggers and Reset Your System: *The Inflammation Spectrum*
Dr. Will Cole

Nutritional Medicine, *Second Edition*
Alan R. Gaby, M.D.

The Lyme Solution: *A 5-Part Plan to Fight the Inflammatory Auto-Immune Response and Beat Lyme Disease*
Darin Ingels, ND, FAAEM

Safe Uses of Cortisol
William Mc K. Jefferies

Toxic: *Heal Your Body from Mold Toxicity, Lyme Disease, Multiple Chemical Sensitivities, and Chronic Environmental Illness*
Neil Nathan, M.D.

Toxic Legacy: *How The Weed Killer Glyphosate Is Destroying Our Health And The Environment*
Stephanie Seneff, PhD

New Paradigms in Lyme Disease Treatment
Connie Strasheim

ACKNOWLEDGMENTS

These are the humans that deserve some serious acknowledgment.

First ...

My sister for making sure I stayed alive and safe when I was a kid.

My best friend, Rina, for making sure I stayed alive and sane as an adult.

And now, I guess the best way to tackle the rest of this is by going in chronological order from when I became an NP.

Dr. Ron Ben Meir who I worked with when I first came out of school. The time between patients was priceless, brother.

PA Ed Rakler for taking a chance on a new hire. Your clinic inspired me to open up EG Healthcare.

Dr. Steven G (I can't spell your name; it's just not happening). You're a little out there, and I will never agree with you on many topics, but you cured my wife and started us on the path that brought us to this book.

To Dr. Frank Scafuri, who took me under his wing for no good reason other than that is just the kind of guy he is.

To the doctors that retired and sold me their pediatric practices: Dr. Helena Gottlieb, Dr. Joel Stakofsky, and Dr. Vijay Chandrakant. Thank you for entrusting me with your patients.

To Dr. Sid Prakash, Dr. Mohammed Zgheib, Dr. Ana Mendez, Dr. Anu Sampat, and Dr. Rumana Sultana, for always answering a text about a patient who needs your expertise. It takes a village.

To Jason and Chris for always helping me network and having unnecessary lunches and dinners.

To Dr. Pat Tooker, who said yes on first sight and magically turned me into "Professor LaMandre."

To Phil Mancuso, who took a risk by putting an outsider on the board (and then doubled down and made me co-chair), and John Demoleas, Michael Caridi, and Dr. Ardolic for supporting the decision.

Dr. Stephen Ferrara for putting up with my bull-in-a-china-shop shenanigans at the NPA.

Dr. Sal Volpe and the PPS—even though I argue with you just about every time I see you, your programs helped elevate EG Healthcare and make it the amazing Primary Care Practice that it is (and P.S. I'm still going to keep arguing with you).

Jose and Rosa Cruz, Cirenia Peralta, Jorge Moreno, Marco Benavides, Ofer Noga, and Adolfo De La Pena for keeping the bricks and mortar of EG running. Without you, it would be too hot, too cold, too wet, too dark, and our computers would crash.

To Phil Black, my annoying mentor, who keeps telling me I'm thinking too small every time I think big. To Ying, for keeping my taxes on point; to Tony for keeping my books on point; and to Barry Ceplowitz and his team for ensuring that my crazy ideas don't break any rules or laws.

To Molly Mahoney, who took The Knew Method to the next level. You started off as my social media guru and became a great friend.

To Matt, my web designer and so much more, who turns every one of my insane ideas into a working website and then redoes it again, and again, and again.

To the Nurse Practitioners who work at EG for being so amazing at your craft and ensuring that EG's reputation stays intact as I work on all the other projects in my head (Diana Macaulay, Rachel Lucente, Gwen Hernandez and Dana Materia).

To my scribes in India, Hari and Shatki. Who would ever have imagined that I would meet two women all the way in India who would become my friends and inspire me to open a medical scribe company? I appreciate the risks you took and the hard work you do.

NOW, FOR SOME VANITY ACKNOWLEDGMENTS ...

My barber, Johnny, for keeping my hair fresh and agreeing to meet me at ungodly hours of the morning because my schedule is insane.

Daniel Friedman for creating suits that don't conform to gender rules. Turns out even my suits are non-conformists. What you do for people's self-image borders on magical.

Barbara Sammarco for keeping me fit despite all my injuries. Our training sessions have become therapy sessions. I should pay you double.

SAVING THE BEST FOR LAST ...

The EG TEAM—a collection of women from all walks of life who get the mission and know what it takes. They have created a culture at EG of accountability, integrity, and intensity. I have to mention my two right hands, Toni Marie, who holds down the fort at EG, and Cayla, who listens to my ideas and figures out how to make them a reality.

One last thing ... for everyone who has ever been in my life—good, bad and indifferent—thank you. I would not be at this exact place, whatever that is, if I hadn't met you.

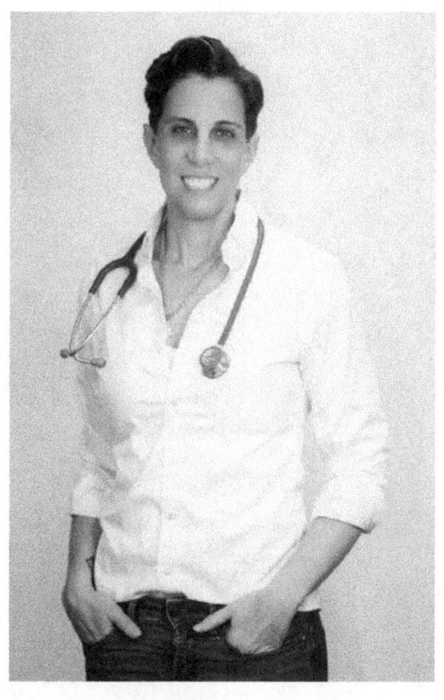

EFRAT LAMANDRE, PhD, FNP-C is a Medical Entrepreneur. She sees a problem, finds the solution, and creates a system around it. In addition to creating The Knew Method, she has established EG Healthcare, EG Prep and Hawk Scribes which are all companies designed to solve various issues in the healthcare industry. When she is not working (and even when she is) she spends time with her amazing wife and together they raise three children and eight cats (that number may have increased since the writing of this sentence. The cats, not the kids).